A Systematic Approach to Assessment and Evaluation of Nursing Programs

A Systematic Approach to Assessment and Evaluation of Nursing Programs

Edited by:
Marilyn H. Oermann, PhD, RN, FAAN, ANEF

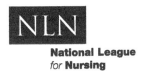

National League
for **Nursing**

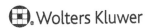

Philadelphia • Baltimore • New York • London
Buenos Aires • Hong Kong • Sydney • Tokyo

Executive Editor: Sherry Dickinson
Product Development Editor: Meredith L. Brittain
Editorial Assistant: Dan Reilly
Production Project Manager: Marian Bellus
Design Coordinator: Terry Mallon
Illustration Coordinator: Jennifer Clements
Manufacturing Coordinator: Karin Duffield
Marketing Manager: Todd McQueston

Oermann, M.H. (2017). *A Systematic Approach to Assessment and Evaluation of Nursing Programs.* Washington, DC: National League for Nursing.

9 8 7 6 5 4 3 2 1

Printed in the United States of America

Library of Congress Cataloging-in-Publication Data

Names: Oermann, Marilyn H., editor. | National League for Nursing, issuing
   body.
Title: A systematic approach to assessment and evaluation of nursing programs
   / edited by Marilyn H. Oermann.
Description: [Washington, D.C.] : NLN, National League for Nursing ;
   Philadelphia : Wolters Kluwer, [2017] | Includes bibliographical
   references.
Identifiers: LCCN 2016002296 | ISBN 9781934758250 (alk. paper)
Subjects: | MESH: Education, Nursing–organization & administration | Program
   Evaluation | Schools, Nursing–organization & administration | Curriculum
   | United States
Classification: LCC RT90 | NLM WY 18 | DDC 610.73071/1–dc23
LC record available at http://lccn.loc.gov/2016002296

www.LWW.com   www.NLN.org

About the Editor

Marilyn H. Oermann, PhD, RN, FAAN, ANEF, is the Thelma M. Ingles Professor of Nursing and Director of Evaluation and Educational Research at Duke University School of Nursing, Durham, North Carolina. She is the Editor-in-Chief of *Nurse Educator* and the *Journal of Nursing Care Quality*. Dr. Oermann is the author/co-author of 17 books, more than 150 articles in peer-reviewed journals, and many other types of publications. Her current books are *Evaluation and Testing in Nursing Education* (4th ed.); *Writing for Publication in Nursing* (3rd ed.); *Teaching in Nursing and Role of the Educator: The Complete Guide to Best Practice in Teaching, Evaluation, and Curriculum Development;* and *Clinical Teaching Strategies in Nursing* (4th ed.). 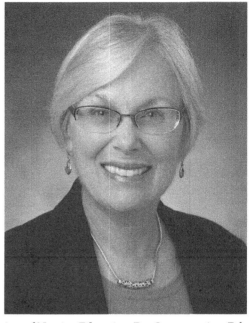 She edited six volumes of the *Annual Review of Nursing Education*. Dr. Oermann is a Fellow in the American Academy of Nursing and the National League for Nursing (NLN) Academy of Nursing Education. She received the NLN Award for Excellence in Nursing Education Research and the Sigma Theta Tau International Elizabeth Russell Belford Award for Excellence in Education.

About the Contributors

Thomas Christenbery, PhD, RN, CNE, is an Associate Professor at Vanderbilt University School of Nursing, Nashville, Tennessee. He serves as the Director of Program Evaluation in the School. In addition to program evaluation, his publications and research concentration include best practices in nursing education and evidence-based practice. Dr. Christenbery serves as a mentor for staff nurses in the Evidence-based Practice Fellowship Program at Vanderbilt University Medical Center. He is the faculty advisor for Vanderbilt's chapter of the American Assembly of Men in Nursing.

Karen H. Frith, PhD, RN, NEA-BC, is Professor of Nursing and Associate Dean for Undergraduate Programs in the College of Nursing, The University of Alabama in Huntsville, Huntsville, Alabama. She is board certified as Nurse Executive, Advanced by the American Nurses Credentialing Center. In her prior position at Georgia College & State University, she served as a department chair with responsibilities for undergraduate and graduate courses. Dr. Frith has a notable scholarship record, with over 30 peer-reviewed journal articles and two books. She serves on review boards for seven journals and is a member of several professional organizations including Sigma Theta Tau International Honor Society of Nursing (Beta Phi Chapter), the American Organization of Nurse Executives, and the Southern Nursing Research Society.

Nelda Godfrey, PhD, ACNS-BC, FAAN, is Associate Dean for Undergraduate Programs and Clinical Professor at the University of Kansas School of Nursing, Kansas City, Kansas. Her scholarly interests include organizational change and culture change, identity formation in health care professionals, and clinical and professional ethics. She has taught leadership and management in graduate and undergraduate education for more than 20 years, and has led substantive organizational change in two academic settings. A champion of curriculum alignment and concept-based learning, Dr. Godfrey is a frequent speaker on these topics, consulting with associate degree and baccalaureate schools throughout the United States.

Judith A. Halstead, PhD, RN, FAAN, ANEF, is Executive Director of the National League for Nursing (NLN) Commission for Nursing Education Accreditation in Washington, DC, a position she has held since July 2014. She has over 35 years of experience in nursing education, with expertise in online education, nurse educator competencies, and evidence-based teaching in nursing. She is co-editor of the widely referenced book, *Teaching in Nursing: A Guide for Faculty*. Dr. Halstead is the recipient of numerous awards including the MNRS Advancement of Science Award for the Nursing Education Research Section and Sigma Theta Tau International Elizabeth Russell Belford Excellence in Education Award. She is a fellow in the NLN Academy of Nursing Education and American Academy of Nursing, and served as the president of the NLN from 2011 to 2013.

Jayalakshmi Jambunathan, PhD, RN, is a Distinguished Professor, Assistant Dean, and Director of Research and Evaluation at the University of Wisconsin, Oshkosh, Wisconsin. She has over 30 years of teaching experience in nursing education including several years in program evaluation, curriculum planning, and assessment of student learning outcomes. Her scholarly interests include academic, clinical, and cross-cultural research focusing on nursing education and evidence-based practice. She is the recipient of several university awards including the Curwood Inc. Endowed Professorship, John F. Kerrigan International Endowed Professorship, Edward M. Penson Distinguished Teaching Award, John McHaughton Rosebush Professorship, and Barbara Sniffen Service awards. She has authored and co-authored multiple publications with faculty and students, and has presented her work at regional, national, and international arenas.

Sharon Kumm, MN, MS, CNE, is a Clinical Associate Professor at the University of Kansas School of Nursing, Kansas City, Kansas, where she has taught for over 20 years. Her scholarly work focuses on curriculum development and technology to enhance student learning. She chaired the taskforce for curriculum revision, which led to the development of a standards-driven, concept-based curriculum with a competency-based clinical for the undergraduate nursing program. She also chaired the taskforce that resulted in the nursing program being designated as an NLN Center of Excellence. Ms. Kumm is a Health Information Technology Scholar and an NLN-certified nurse educator.

Lynne Porter Lewallen, PhD, RN, CNE, ANEF, is Professor and Assistant Dean for Academic Affairs in the School of Nursing at the University of North Carolina at Greensboro, Greensboro, North Carolina. She is an accreditation site visitor and team chair, and has experience speaking and consulting about program evaluation. Her research interests include health promotion in pregnancy and prenatal care, and clinical evaluation in nursing education. Dr. Lewallen serves on the NLN Research Review Panel and Editorial Board of *Nursing Education Perspectives*.

Joan Such Lockhart, PhD, RN, CORLN, AOCN, CNE, FAAN, ANEF, is a tenured clinical professor and MSN Nursing Education Program Coordinator at Duquesne University School of Nursing, Pittsburgh, Pennsylvania. As the former Associate Dean for Academic Affairs, she co-chaired the University's Academic Learning Outcomes Assessment Committee, led the school's program evaluation processes, and was instrumental in its successful accreditation and NLN Center of Excellence recognitions. Her scholarship mirrors her expertise in oncology, nursing professional development, and academic education with a focus on culturally diverse and vulnerable populations. Dr. Lockhart is a fellow in the American Academy of Nursing and NLN Academy of Nursing Education, serves as the Associate Editor for the *Journal of Continuing Education in Nursing* and *ORL - Head and Neck Nursing*, and is on the editorial board of *Nurse Educator*. She recently authored *Nursing Professional Development for Clinical Educators* for the Oncology Nursing Society.

Suzanne Marnocha, PhD, RN, CCRN, ret., is the Curler Endowed Professor of Health Sciences and Assistant Dean and Pre-Licensure Director, College of Nursing, University of Wisconsin Oshkosh, Oshkosh, Wisconsin. She directs Wisconsin's largest Bachelor of

Science in Nursing program and is a nurse researcher who regularly presents and publishes her work. She has been recognized by the Wisconsin Nurses Association with the 100 Faces of Nursing award. In addition to her Curler Endowed Professorship for Health Sciences, she received the Edward M. Penson Faculty Award from the University of Wisconsin Oshkosh. Dr. Marnocha is the President-Elect for the Association for Nurse Educators of Wisconsin and is actively engaged as a nursing leader in the community by serving on a large elder care community board of directors and a church leadership advisory team.

Melinda G. Oberleitner, DNS, RN, is Associate Dean, College of Nursing and Allied Health Professions, and a Professor in the Department of Nursing at the University of Louisiana at Lafayette, Lafayette, Louisiana. She holds the SLEMCO/BORSF Endowed Professorship in Nursing. Dr. Oberleitner has extensive experience in nursing education and academic program administration, and has taught at the undergraduate and graduate levels for over 30 years. Her teaching, scholarly publications, presentations, and funded grants have focused on nursing leadership and management, oncology nursing, and nursing education. In 2015, Dr. Oberleitner was selected as an American Association of Colleges of Nursing/Wharton Executive Nurse Leadership Fellow at the Wharton School of the University of Pennsylvania.

Karen J. Saewert, PhD, RN, CPHQ, CNE, ANEF, is a Clinical Professor and Senior Director for Academic Innovation in the College of Nursing & Health Innovation at Arizona State University, Phoenix, Arizona. Her work focuses on assessment and evaluation in support of teaching and learning excellence, quality assessment, delivery of innovative nontraditional curricula, outcomes measurement and systems development, and interprofessional health professions education and practice. Dr. Saewert serves as Evaluation Lead for the statewide Arizona Nexus, one of eight "pioneer" Nexus Innovations Incubator team sites within the Nexus Innovations Network of the National Center for Interprofessional Practice and Education. She is a Certified Professional in Healthcare Quality and an NLN-certified nurse educator. Dr. Saewert is a Fellow of the NLN Academy of Nursing Education.

Teresa Shellenbarger, PhD, RN, CNE, ANEF, is a Professor in the Department of Nursing and Allied Health Professions, Indiana University of Pennsylvania, Indiana, Pennsylvania. She has been a nurse educator for more than 25 years and has taught in multiple levels of nursing education. An accomplished author, researcher, and nursing leader, Dr. Shellenbarger has expertise in program development, assessment and evaluation, innovative teaching strategies, faculty role development, and technology use in education. She is an NLN-certified nurse educator and was inducted as an inaugural fellow in the NLN Academy of Nursing Education.

Theresa M. "Terry" Valiga, EdD, RN, CNE, FAAN, ANEF, is a Professor at Duke University School of Nursing, Durham, North Carolina, where she also serves as the Director of the School's Institute for Educational Excellence and Chair of the Division of Systems and Analytics. Immediately prior to her appointment at Duke, she served as the Chief Program Officer at the NLN. She has published extensively on a variety of leadership and education-related topics, co-authored five books, served on governing boards of several national organizations, presented papers and workshops at national and international conferences, and served as a consultant to many schools of nursing throughout the United States and in other countries. Dr. Valiga has received prestigious national awards including Sigma Theta Tau's Elizabeth Russell Belford Founders Award for Excellence in Nursing Education and the NLN's Outstanding Leadership in Nursing Education Award. She is a Fellow of the Academy of Nursing Education and American Academy of Nursing.

Foreword

The fourth core value of the National League for Nursing (NLN) is Excellence, which we define as "co-creating and implementing transformative strategies with daring ingenuity." This book, edited by Marilyn H. Oermann, is a fine example of the implementation of this value. The co-creating happens as the editor, in partnership with other authors, navigates the field of formative and summative evaluation for schools of nursing. This develops the potential guided implementation and documented outcomes of program decision-making at schools of nursing throughout the United States and the global community.

As a significant missing piece of the puzzle for successful accreditation, steps to deliver ongoing formative and summative evaluation for nursing programs represent truly transformative strategies. The strategies offered in this book, itemized in detail by expert faculty, can be used to change the culture for nursing programs attempting to seek successful accreditation. For programs that have already achieved accreditation, the strategies presented here will offer options for ongoing systematic assessment and evaluation that are based on evidence. We promote evidence-based nursing practice but do not yet have evidence-based nursing education programs. Our students deserve a culture of nursing school programs built on evidence, one that is vital for the successful transformation of our health care system and the well-being of our patients.

Colleagues, you will find the daring ingenuity of excellence in each of these chapters. Along with the accreditation of nursing programs, the chapters explore program evaluation models, the development of systematic program evaluation plans for schools of nursing, the assessment of online courses and programs, the evaluation of specific program types, and the successful management of organizational change. You will find much more in these pages for a subject that has never been addressed under one cover for the nursing community.

This textbook touches the foundation of quality nursing education and will be useful for faculty and graduate students across all types of nursing programs. So, I am pleased to bring you Excellence, from this book's outstanding editor, Dr. Oermann, and the incredible authors, all dedicated to transforming nursing education and fulfilling the mission of the NLN: The NLN promotes excellence in nursing education to build a strong and diverse nursing workforce to advance the health of the nation and global community.

Beverly Malone, PhD, RN, FAAN
CEO
National League for Nursing

Preface

Program evaluation is a systematic process of collecting data for making decisions about a nursing program and judging its value. With the need to offer high-quality nursing programs and continued growth of new programs and delivery methods, systematic and ongoing program evaluation is critical across all schools of nursing and levels of education. Program evaluation not only provides data for decision-making within an organization but also for accreditation.

The focus of this book is on assessment and evaluation of nursing programs, not the evaluation of individual students and their learning. The book provides under one cover the concepts that nurse educators should understand to engage in program evaluation and accreditation, and includes examples, guidelines, and practical strategies for "getting it done." The book was written for nurse educators, administrators, and others involved in program evaluation in all types of nursing programs and for nursing students in graduate courses that include program evaluation. Nurse educators in clinical settings who are responsible for developing and evaluating educational programs also may find the book helpful.

Chapter 1 provides an overview of assessment and evaluation, describes the purposes of program evaluation, and examines differences between formative and summative evaluation. Because the evaluation needs to provide the "right" information to make decisions about the program and to answer faculty, administrator, and other stakeholder questions, the process should be systematic, well planned, and ongoing. The steps in program evaluation are described in this chapter.

Chapter 2 explores general models and perspectives to consider when planning for program assessment and evaluation. The process of evaluation should lead to the use of findings by a variety of stakeholders. For this to occur, program evaluation must be understandable, relevant, meaningful, credible, and focused on actions or decisions leading to program- and organization-level learning and improvement. Optimal program evaluation is accomplished through assigning value to evaluation, making sound evaluative judgments, putting evaluation principles into practice, and meeting evaluation standards.

Faculty in schools of nursing spend a great deal of time designing the curriculum, implementing it in ways that engage the learner, and evaluating what students have learned as a result of those experiences. Efforts to evaluate the entire curriculum, however, are often overlooked, not approached in a systematic way, and incomplete. Chapter 3 addresses the purposes of, and ways to approach, curriculum evaluation; relates this activity to the overall program evaluation; and clarifies the role of faculty in the curriculum development, evaluation, and revision process.

Meaningful program evaluation results are dependent on well thought-out, relevant evaluation questions. These questions are often based on information needed for accreditation and to address concerns of key stakeholders. Chapter 4 provides guidelines for writing good evaluation questions, creating and selecting high-quality survey questions, and identifying appropriate indicators. Examples of various types of program evaluation questions are provided. This chapter contains the information you need to prepare your own surveys and other tools for program evaluation.

Systematic program evaluation is critical for program improvement as well as adherence to regulatory and accreditation standards. Chapter 5 discusses the rationale for program evaluation and how to get started in creating a program evaluation plan or revising an existing plan. Areas to include in a plan are described, and samples of actual evaluation plans from two nursing programs are used to illustrate strategies to evaluate selected criteria.

The evaluation plan specifies the types of data to collect for program evaluation. Faculty rely on systematically collected quality data to make good decisions about their nursing program. Chapter 6 provides an overview of data and data sources frequently used in nursing program evaluation. Psychometric considerations of reliability and validity, internal and external factors that have an impact on data quality, and types and forms of data collection approaches, including quantitative and qualitative, are described in the chapter. Also included are innovative strategies for using technology to assist in gathering program evaluation data.

Chapter 7 describes the purpose of higher education (postsecondary) accreditation in the United States, types of accreditation, and usual program elements represented in accreditation standards for nursing education. The chapter also provides an overview of the accreditation process and explains the relationships among program evaluation, continuous quality improvement, and the accreditation process.

The process of accreditation is rigorous, and preparing for accreditation can be overwhelming. Chapter 8 offers specific guidelines and helpful tips in preparing for the accreditation process, including writing the self-study. A sample site visit schedule and resource room guide, and other materials developed by a school to guide its preparation for accreditation and the site visit, are included in the chapter and Appendix C.

Assessment of online courses and programs is an integral part of a nursing program's systematic program evaluation plan. Regardless of the level of course or academic degree, guidelines and approaches have been developed that can promote effective evaluation. Chapter 9 addresses evaluating online courses, establishing benchmarks for program success, and assessing the quality of courses and programs using valid and reliable tools. In addition, the chapter discusses the issues related to nursing courses and programs offered in other states and their impact on evaluation and accreditation.

Chapter 10 focuses on specific types of nursing programs: RN to BSN, accelerated second career, nurse practitioner, nurse anesthetist, and doctoral nursing programs. These programs have unique assessment needs. The chapter examines areas important to evaluate in addition to the typical components of program evaluation.

Change is a reality in all organizations, with many organizations having continual change. Some organizations are more successful than others in transitioning and successfully managing change. Chapter 11 explores change and leadership theories that are particularly useful in academic environments, the change process itself and factors that can impede or foster change, a systems approach to evaluation, making organizational decisions based on assessment and evaluation data, considerations in maximizing stakeholder investment in the change process, and strategies for balancing resources and costs when implementing organizational change.

Thank you to the NLN for identifying the need for a book that addresses program evaluation in nursing. The chapter authors deserve a special acknowledgment for sharing their expertise, helpful tips, and sample materials with readers, and for their enthusiasm about this book. We hope that you find the book valuable as you engage in assessment and evaluation of your nursing program.

Marilyn H. Oermann, PhD, RN, FAAN, ANEF
Thelma M. Ingles Professor of Nursing
Director of Evaluation and Educational Research
Duke University School of Nursing
Durham, North Carolina

Contents

About the Editor   v

About the Contributors   vi

Foreword   x

Preface   xi

CHAPTER 1   **Program Evaluation: An Introduction**   1
Marilyn H. Oermann, PhD, RN, FAAN, ANEF

CHAPTER 2   **Program Evaluation Perspectives and Models**   7
Karen J. Saewert, PhD, RN, CPHQ, CNE, ANEF

CHAPTER 3   **Curriculum Evaluation**   19
Theresa M. "Terry" Valiga, EdD, RN, CNE, FAAN, ANEF

CHAPTER 4   **Formulating Evaluation Questions**   29
Thomas Christenbery, PhD, RN, CNE

CHAPTER 5   **Developing a Systematic Program Evaluation Plan for a School of Nursing**   45
Lynne Porter Lewallen, PhD, RN, CNE, ANEF

CHAPTER 6   **Ensuring Quality of Evaluation Data**   59
Teresa Shellenbarger, PhD, RN, CNE, ANEF

CHAPTER 7   **The Accreditation Process in Nursing Education**   79
Judith A. Halstead, PhD, RN, FAAN, ANEF

CHAPTER 8   **Program Evaluation: Getting it Done in Your School of Nursing**   93
Suzanne Marnocha, PhD, RN, CCRN, ret. and Jayalakshmi Jambunathan, PhD, RN

CHAPTER 9   **Assessment of Online Courses and Programs**   103
Karen H. Frith, PhD, RN, NEA-BC

CHAPTER 10   **Evaluation of Specific Program Types and Impact on Program Assessment and Evaluation**   119
Joan Such Lockhart, PhD, RN, CORLN, AOCN, CNE, FAAN, ANEF and Melinda G. Oberleitner, DNS, RN

CHAPTER 11   **Managing Organizational Change Effectively**   135
Sharon Kumm, MN, MS, CNE and
Nelda Godfrey, PhD, ACNS-BC, FAAN

Appendix A. Examples of Completed Evaluation Plans   149
Appendix B. Joint Committee on Standards for Educational Evaluation (JCSEE) Program Evaluation Standards Statements   167
Appendix C. Sample Site Visit Schedule and Resource Room Guide   171

List of Figures and Tables

LIST OF FIGURES

Figure 2.1   Framework for Program Evaluation   15

Figure 8.1   A Resource Room Should be Well Lit and Quiet, with a Large Desk   99

Figure 8.2   Resource Room Documents Organization   100

Figure 11.1   Institutional Resources and Costs   143

LIST OF TABLES

Table 2.1   Reframed Evaluation Assumptions   8

Table 2.2   Overview of Selected Models for Program Evaluation   12

Table 4.1   Characteristics of Survey Questions   33

Table 4.2   Types of Closed-Ended Questions   36

Table 6.1   Comparison of Data Collection Methods   66

Table 7.1   Accreditation Standards for ACEN, CCNE, and NLN CNEA   85

Table 9.1   Comparison of C-RAC, ACEN, and CCNE Standards
for Accreditation for Distance Education Programs 105

Table 9.2   Sample Plan for Measuring Quality in Distance Education
Courses and Programs   112

Table 11.1   Methods to Engage Stakeholders   139

Table 11.2   Techniques and Tools Useful in Each Stage of Change Process   141

Table A.1   Completed Evaluation Plans for Faculty and Student Participation in
Program Governance   150

Table A.2   Completed Evaluation Plans for Faculty Expertise Criterion   154

Table A.3   Completed Evaluation Plans for Assessment of Student Complaints   157

Table A.4   Completed Evaluation Plans for Assessment of Curriculum by
Faculty   159

Table A.5   Completed Evaluation Plans for Assessment of Physical Resources   161

Table A.6   Completed Evaluation Plans for Graduate Satisfaction Criterion   164

Table C.1   Day One Site Visit Schedule   172

Table C.2   Resource Room Guide Examples   174

1

Program Evaluation:
An Introduction

Marilyn H. Oermann, PhD, RN, FAAN, ANEF

Program evaluation is a systematic process of collecting data for making decisions about a nursing program and judging its value. Evaluation is essential to identify the needs within the school, provide feedback while a program is being developed, and establish the program's effectiveness following its completion. With evaluation that is done continuously, faculty, administrators, and other stakeholders learn what is working well in their nursing program and where changes are needed to improve quality. This chapter provides a brief overview of program evaluation and its importance in nursing education.

ASSESSMENT, EVALUATION, AND MEASUREMENT

Evaluation is essential for answering questions about the effectiveness of the program in promoting students' learning and preparing them for their future roles, quality of the educational experiences, satisfaction of students and others with the program, and program improvements. Evaluation allows faculty, administrators, and other stakeholders—people or groups invested in the program—to collect data and use those data for making informed decisions that will improve program quality. Without evaluation, decisions may be made based on tradition or what individuals and groups *think* will work best. With the high cost of nursing education and limited time for students to acquire the knowledge, skills, and values that they need for practice, decisions about the curriculum, instruction, students, faculty, resources, and other areas need to be made carefully and be based on sound information.

Evaluation is integral to developing a high-quality nursing program and maintaining its quality. It cannot be an "add on" or done only for accreditation purposes: It has to be part of the culture of the school of nursing. Evaluation should be done routinely when faculty, administrators, and others need to make an educational decision; that decision should be based on relevant data. Evaluation also promotes accountability: Data collected

1

through a systematic evaluation document outcomes of the program and its successes, and reveal areas in need of improvement.

Terms such as *assessment, evaluation,* and *measurement* are sometimes used interchangeably, but there are differences that readers should be aware of. Assessment is the process of obtaining information to use for making educational decisions (Nitko & Brookhart, 2011; Oermann & Gaberson, 2014). Many strategies are available for collecting information related to an educational program including tests; surveys of students, faculty, and other stakeholders; focus groups; interviews; observations; rating scales; e-portfolios; and analyses of capstone and other end-of-program projects, among others. The type of strategy needs to be appropriate for the purpose and questions to be answered so that it provides the "right" information. Nitko and Brookhart (2011) emphasized the need to use multiple strategies for assessment.

Evaluation is the process of making a judgment as to value and worth based on the information. Scriven (2013) defined evaluation as the process of determining or declaring the merit, worth, or significance of a product or entity (p. 170). Answering questions such as these requires a value judgment: (1) How *well* did students perform on the comprehensive tests prior to and following the course revision?; (2) What is the *effectiveness* of the on-campus intensive experience in developing students' competencies in interprofessional collaboration?; and (3) How *satisfied* are students with the program? While assessment is the process of obtaining information, when judgments are made about value and worth, the process has extended to evaluation.

Mark and Henry (2013) expanded this view of evaluation. They suggested that there were four purposes of evaluation in educational settings: (1) for an overall assessment and judgment as to merit and worth, with evaluation supporting that judgment; (2) for program and organizational improvement, with evaluation pointing to needed changes in the program and organization; (3) for accountability and oversight, with evaluation providing information about the program's compliance with standards and mandates; and (4) for knowledge development, with the goal of evaluation to improve understanding, for example, of a health care issue or new approaches to teaching that might be used in the program.

Measurement is not the same as assessment or evaluation. Measurement involves using scores or numbers to represent an outcome or characteristic. Mean scores on a survey of a course or program, test scores, and scales that indicate the quality of a student's performance in a skills laboratory are examples of measurements.

In this book, we use the term *evaluation* broadly to include information collected in an assessment of the program and the resulting judgments of value and worth. Those judgments lead faculty, administrators, and other stakeholders to decisions about needed improvements in the program or to maintain the program as is.

PURPOSES OF PROGRAM EVALUATION

There are many reasons to engage in program evaluation. All too often, faculty and administrators think of program evaluation in terms of accreditation. While one of the purposes of program evaluation is to confirm that accreditation standards are met, this is only one purpose.

Through program evaluation, faculty can determine if students are achieving the outcomes of the program as well as the intended knowledge and competencies. Assessment and evaluation are essential components of nursing courses, but program evaluation examines students' achievement and professional development across courses as they progress through the program.

Program evaluation enables schools of nursing to identify the needs within the school, the institution in which it is housed, and the community. Using this information, faculty and administrators may decide to develop a new course or program, revise current ones, begin or continue an initiative in the school, vary instructional methods, seek new clinical sites, or develop new resources.

Program evaluation also provides data for modifying processes to improve efficiency and better meet student and other stakeholder needs. The information obtained through an evaluation can help faculty and administrators examine day-to-day processes in the program to assess if they are working well and identify areas and practices in need of improvement. Questions such as whether the clinical placement process is effective and what issues occur with arranging placements for students can be answered through a systematic evaluation, uncovering issues and leading to recommendations to improve processes.

Internal and External Evaluation Focus

Another way to think about the purposes of program evaluation is that they can be internal or external. Evaluation for internal purposes is not required by an accrediting body but is done within the school to answer questions of faculty, administrators, and others about various aspects of the program. Surveying students about their satisfaction with the simulation laboratory and adjunct faculty about the value of their orientation are examples of program evaluation done for internal reasons. Typically, the goal of these evaluations is to make program improvements.

In contrast, external reasons are to verify that the nursing program meets requirements and standards of the parent institution within which it is housed, the state board of nursing, and the national nursing accrediting bodies. Institutions are accredited by regional accrediting agencies, such as the Southern Association of Colleges and Schools Commission on Colleges, which accredits degree-granting institutions in the Southern states. Accreditation at the institutional level documents that the community college, college, or university in which the nursing program is housed meets the standards of the accrediting agency. Program evaluation provides data about the nursing unit as part of the institution's accreditation. The evaluation process also verifies that a program meets the state board of nursing requirements as an approved program within the state and the standards for nursing program accreditation through the Commission on Collegiate Nursing Education, the Accreditation Commission for Education in Nursing, or the National League for Nursing Commission for Nursing Education Accreditation.

FORMATIVE AND SUMMATIVE EVALUATION

Program evaluation is not only done at the end when the program is completed, but also during its development to answer specific evaluation questions. Formative evaluation examines the program and its components while they are being developed and implemented. Formative data are reported back to faculty and administrators to identify and address issues. With this type of evaluation, the information can be used to modify the program to ensure its quality and identify where changes are needed. The following is an example of a question asked during formative evaluation: Is the integration of mental health concepts in the courses being implemented as intended?

Summative evaluation provides evidence of the effectiveness of the program and extent of outcomes achieved by graduates. This type of evaluation is used mainly for determining the quality of the program and whether it achieves its mission, goals, and outcomes (Story et al., 2010). Summative evaluation takes place after the program is completed and implemented. The following are examples of questions for guiding summative evaluation: Are students achieving the outcomes of the program? What is the impact on students? What are the costs? What resources are needed? Data from summative evaluation not only determine outcomes but also provide information for subsequent program improvement. Typically, summative data include information such as student scores on standardized tests, scores on end-of-program surveys, National Council Licensure Examination (NCLEX) and certification first-time pass rates, employment rates, and similar measures. Interviews and focus groups with stakeholders also may serve as summative data if the questions are intended to learn about participant responses to different experiences in the program and outcomes that have been achieved (Spaulding, 2014).

STEPS IN PROGRAM EVALUATION

There are many theoretical frameworks and perspectives of evaluation and program evaluation. Some of these are discussed in a later chapter. Across these frameworks and perspectives, one constant is that program evaluation is a systematic and planned process. This is critical because the evaluation needs to provide the "right" information to make decisions about the program and to answer faculty, administrator, and other stakeholder questions.

Identify Purpose of Evaluation

The evaluation process begins by identifying its purpose (Box 1.1). The evaluation may be comprehensive and broad, for example, evaluating outcomes of the program, or narrow in scope, such as determining the effectiveness of a peer-alumni tutoring program. The purpose of the evaluation and scope also influences the extent of the resources (time, costs) needed to complete the evaluation. An evaluation that is narrow and more focused generally requires less time to do and fewer resources.

BOX 1.1

Steps in Program Evaluation

1. Identify purpose of the evaluation.
2. Develop questions to be answered through evaluation.
3. Design the evaluation.
4. Collect and analyze the evaluation data.
5. Report findings and use for program improvement, if indicated.

Develop Questions to be Answered through Evaluation

Considering the purpose of the evaluation, the next step is to identify the questions to be answered. An example of a question related to program outcomes is: What is the first-time pass rate on the NCLEX for graduates of the BSN program? To examine the effectiveness of the tutoring program, a question might be: Do students who participate in peer-alumni tutoring achieve passing grades in their pathophysiology course, and are they satisfied with the tutoring program? The evaluation is designed and implemented to answer those questions. For that reason, the evaluation questions are critical: They "determine and constrict everything in the evaluation process that comes with it" (Chelimsky, 2013, p. 269).

Design the Evaluation

The evaluation questions guide the design of the evaluation and types of data collected. This is the step in which the faculty or other evaluators identify the information needed to answer their questions. Some of the data may be available currently in the program; if not, tools and other strategies will need to be identified to provide the essential data. This step in the evaluation process also includes deciding on the time frame for data collection. For example, to assess the effectiveness of the peer-alumni tutoring program, intended to promote success in the pathophysiology course, grades in the course and the findings from a survey of students' satisfaction with the tutoring would be examined at the end of the course. These data might be collected only at this one point in time. However, to assess students' perceptions of their achievement of program outcomes and satisfaction with the program, data might be collected at the end of the program and from alumni one year postgraduation.

Collect and Analyze Evaluation Data

The next step is to collect and analyze the data. The evaluation plan should specify the expected levels of performance and the expected criteria to be achieved, which are used to interpret the data. For example, for the broad question on first-time pass rate, the expected criterion might be for 90% of graduates to pass the NCLEX the first time taken. For peer-alumni tutoring, the criterion might be that 95% of the students who complete all tutoring sessions pass the pathophysiology course and 85% report satisfaction with the tutoring on a survey. The criteria guide the faculty and others in interpreting the data and ascribing meaning to the information collected in the evaluation.

Report Findings and Use for Program Improvement, if Indicated

The findings from program evaluation need to be reported to those who can use the information for making decisions. Boland (2015) recommended that a common repository be created to ensure that the evaluation data are collected and analyzed on a cyclical basis and are available for easy retrieval. Evaluation data should be stored electronically, and the information system should allow for displaying the data for specific audiences and needs. The evaluation process involves systematically collecting and analyzing data. Those data, in turn, should be used to make evidence-based changes and improvements in the nursing program (Ellis & Halstead, 2012). Wholey (2013) emphasized that the key is to plan and design evaluations that provide credible and useful information for the school.

SUMMARY

Program evaluation is a systematic process of collecting information about a nursing program for making informed decisions. Through evaluation, faculty, administrators, and others can judge the value and worth of the program and its many components. Evaluation is essential to identify needs within the school, to provide feedback while a program is being developed, and to establish the program's effectiveness following its completion. With evaluation that is done continuously, faculty, administrators, and other stakeholders learn what is working well in their nursing program and where changes are needed to improve quality.

References

Boland, D. L. (2015). Program evaluation. In M. H. Oermann (Ed.), *Teaching in nursing and role of the educator: The complete guide to best practice in teaching, evaluation, and curriculum development* (pp. 275–301). New York: Springer.

Chelimsky, E. (2013). Evaluation purposes, perspectives, and practice. In M. C. Alkin (Ed.), *Evaluation roots: A wider perspective of theorists' views and influences* (pp. 267–282). Los Angeles: Sage.

Ellis, P., & Halstead, J. (2012). Understanding the Commission on Collegiate Nursing Education accreditation process and the continuous improvement progress report. *Journal of Professional Nursing, 28,* 18–26.

Mark, M. M., & Henry, G. T. (2013). Multiple routes: Evaluation, assisted sensemaking, and pathways to betterment. In M. C. Alkin (Ed.), *Evaluation roots: A wider perspective of theorists' views and influences* (pp. 144–156). Los Angeles: Sage.

Nitko, A. J., & Brookhart, S. M. (2011). *Educational assessment of students* (6th ed.). Upper Saddle River, NJ: Pearson Education.

Oermann, M. H., & Gaberson, K. B. (2014). *Evaluation and testing in nursing education* (4th ed.). New York: Springer.

Scriven, M. (2013). Conceptual revolutions in evaluation: Past, present, and future. In M. C. Alkin (Ed.), *Evaluation roots: A wider perspective of theorists' views and influences* (pp. 167–179). Los Angeles: Sage.

Spaulding, D.T. (2014). *Program evaluation in practice: Core concepts and examples for discussion and analysis* (2nd ed.). Somerset, NJ: John Wiley & Sons, Inc.

Story, L., Butts, J. B., Bishop, S. B., Green, L., Johnson, K., & Mattison, H. (2010). Innovative strategies for nursing education program evaluation. *Journal of Nursing Education, 49,* 351–354.

Wholey, J. S. (2013). Using evaluation to improve program performance and results. In M. C. Alkin (Ed.), *Evaluation roots: A wider perspective of theorists' views and influences* (pp. 261–265). Los Angeles: Sage.

2

Program Evaluation Perspectives and Models

Karen J. Saewert, PhD, RN, CPHQ, CNE, ANEF

At first glance, program evaluation may appear simple. Even so, entire books, collegiate courses, and doctoral programs focus on program evaluation, theories, methods, and models with roots in sociology, education, public health, and other related fields. Many of the terms, concepts, theories, and frameworks used in educational program evaluation originated from such models. These rudiments of evaluation were adapted to education in response to an increased emphasis on outcomes as a mechanism for public accountability. Assessment and evaluation are used in nursing education and other professional contexts on a daily basis to make decisions.

Nurse educators are evaluators doing evaluation for a reason—there are questions to be answered. Systematic program evaluation, a requirement in nursing education for decades, emphasizes educational effectiveness and public accountability mandated by a broad spectrum of individuals and groups with a stake in the educational process, and contributes to evidence-based nursing education. This chapter builds on the introduction to program assessment and evaluation presented in Chapter 1. It provides an overview of general models to consider when selecting and examining the specific application of assessment and evaluation practices within the contexts addressed in later chapters. Assessment and evaluation prospects, assumptions, and perspectives (e.g., assigning values and making judgments, putting principles into practice, and meeting standards) are also examined in the chapter.

PROSPECT OF EVALUATION

Program assessment and evaluation, ubiquitous in nursing education, vies with other priorities for limited resources at many levels within and across an academic institution and program. Time for evaluation does not just happen (Lewallen, 2015). The contribution of sound evaluative thinking and practice to the achievement of nursing program quality design, delivery, improvements, and outcomes is not without its earned detractors. Integrating standards and criteria required by diverse stakeholder groups into a single

TABLE 2.1	
Reframed Evaluation Assumptions	
Program Evaluation is thought to be	**Program Evaluation can be**
Expensive	Cost-effective
Time-consuming	Strategically timed
Tangential	Integrated
Technical	Accurate
Not inclusive	Engaging
Academic	Practical
Punitive	Helpful
Political	Participatory
Useless	Useful

comprehensive evaluation plan brings challenges. While program evaluation is necessary for understanding and improving educational programs in nursing, it is frequently surrounded by a climate of unease and perplexity (Sarnecky, 1990).

The prospect of evaluation is characterized as troublesome when its methods—perceived as punitive, exclusionary, and adversarial—are counterproductive to using learning from the discovery of evaluation findings for greater program effectiveness (Centers for Disease Control and Prevention [CDC], 1999). Confusion over language further contributes to frustration and resistance to evaluation. Terms used to discuss evaluation concepts often sound ambiguous, are overly technical, and cannot be assumed to mean the same thing to people from different backgrounds (Milstein & Wetterhall, 2000). Establishing a common evaluation vocabulary aids in providing clarity of communication about evaluation and the strategies used; by clarifying evaluation terms, assumptions about evaluation can be reframed to fit an approach designed to be helpful while also engaging interested stakeholders in the process (CDC, 1999) (Table 2.1). Who are these stakeholders? Anyone affected by a program or its evaluation is a *stakeholder* because the findings of the evaluation are used to answer questions and make decisions about the program and its components (Yarbrough, Shulha, Hopson, & Caruthers, 2011).

PROGRAM ASSESSMENT AND EVALUATION: KEY PERSPECTIVES

Assigning Values and Making Judgments

How can program assessment and evaluation be used to better understand and improve education practice? How can we do what we do better? What can be done to make evaluation more understandable and manageable? What strategies can be used to build evaluation literacy, competency, and use in our nursing programs? These and other questions remain timely and timeless. In the late 1990s, the CDC assembled an expert Evaluation Working Group to organize the basic elements of program evaluation and promote use of evaluation standards. The aim was to develop a common understanding of evaluation concepts and advance integration of evaluation in practice.

According to the CDC Evaluation Working Group (CDC, 1999), assigning value and making judgments regarding a program on the basis of evidence requires answering the following questions at the beginning of a program and revisiting them throughout its implementation:

1. What will be evaluated (i.e., what is "the program" and in what context does it exist)?

2. What aspects of the program will be considered when judging program performance?

3. What standards must be reached for the program to be considered successful?

4. What evidence will be used to indicate how the program has performed?

5. What conclusions regarding program performance are justified by comparing the available evidence to the selected standards?

6. How will lessons learned from the inquiry be used to improve program effectiveness?

These questions—asked, answered, and revisited—reinforce an overarching principle: It is important to *understand* the program that is being evaluated; the context and history of the program; the intended purpose of undertaking a program evaluation; and the time, expertise, and resources for conducting a program evaluation (Billings, 2000; Hackbarth & Gall, 2005; Posavac & Carey, 2010; Saewert, 2013; Shadish, Cook, & Leviton, 1991; Spaulding, 2008; Stufflebeam & Shinkfield, 2007).

Putting Principles into Practice

The American Evaluation Association set forth guiding principles for the professional practice of evaluation (American Evaluation Association, 2004). These principles are presented in Box 2.1. However intended, adherence to these principles can implicitly and explicitly impact *any* individual engaged in or affected by program assessment and evaluation activities, making evaluating a nursing program *everyone's responsibility.*

Meeting Standards

Program evaluations are expected to meet specific standards based on five fundamental concepts of evaluation quality recommended by the Joint Committee on Standards for Educational Evaluation: *utility, feasibility, propriety, accuracy,* and *evaluation accountability* (Ruhe & Boudreau, 2013; Saewert, 2013; Stufflebeam & Shinkfield, 2007). The standards based on these fundamental concepts answer the question, "Will this evaluation be effective?" (CDC, 1999). The standards contribute to sound and fair evaluation practices by providing guidelines to follow when deciding among evaluation options.

BOX 2.1

Guiding Principles for the Practice of Evaluation

Systematic inquiry. Evaluators conduct systematic, data-based inquiries about whatever is being evaluated.

Competence. Evaluators provide competent performance to stakeholders.

Integrity and honesty. Evaluators ensure the honesty and integrity of the entire evaluation process.

Respect for people. Evaluators respect the security, dignity, and self-worth of the respondents, program participants, clients, and other stakeholders with whom they interact.

Responsibilities for general and public welfare. Evaluators articulate and take into account the diversity of interests and values that may be related to the general and public welfare.

SOURCE: American Evaluation Association. (2004). *American Evaluation Association Guiding Principles for Evaluators.* http://www.eval.org/p/cm/ld/fid=51.

They guide decisions as to whether a set of evaluative activities are well designed and working to their potential, and are accurate, feasible, and useful (CDC, 1999; Milstein & Wetterhall, 2000).

Utility

If there is no prospect that the findings of an evaluation will be used, it is questionable as to whether the evaluation should be done (Saewert, 2013). The underlying principle of *utility* is that program evaluation should effectively address the information needs of the intended users and other audiences with a right to know, inform program improvement processes, and contribute meaningfully to those persons or groups involved with, or responsible for, implementing the program (CDC, 1999; Ruhe & Boudreau, 2013; Saewert, 2013). The utility standards address identifying those who will be impacted by the evaluation, the amount and type of information collected, the values used in interpreting the findings, and the clarity and timeliness of evaluation reports (Milstein & Wetterhall, 2000). The eight utility standards encompass evaluator credibility, attention to stakeholders, negotiated purposes, explicit values, relevant information, meaningful processes and products, timely and appropriate communicating and reporting, and concern for consequences and influence (Yarbrough, Shulha, Hopson, & Caruthers, 2011).

Feasibility

The *feasibility* standards ensure that the evaluation being conducted is viable and pragmatic (Milstein & Wetterhall, 2000). Program evaluation avoids overly complex methods and employs methods that contribute to evaluation efficiency and cost-effectiveness without disrupting or impairing the program (CDC, 1999; Ruhe & Boudreau, 2013; Saewert, 2013). The feasibility standards address project management, practical procedures, sustainability, and resource use (Yarbrough, Shulha, Hopson, & Caruthers, 2011).

Propriety

Meeting the conditions of the *propriety* standards requires that evaluations be conducted legally, ethically, and with due regard for the welfare of those involved in the evaluation and those affected by the results (CDC, 1999; Milstein & Wetterhall, 2000; Saewert, 2013). The propriety standards support a responsive and inclusive orientation, formal agreements, human rights and respect, clarity and fairness, transparency and disclosure, conflicts of interest, and fiscal responsibility (Yarbrough, Shulha, Hopson, & Caruthers, 2011).

Accuracy

Accuracy refers to the truthfulness, validity and dependability of evaluation findings, and soundness of the interpretations and judgments about program quality. The fundamental concept of *accuracy* and its related standards require that evaluators obtain sound information, analyze it correctly, and report justifiable conclusions (Stufflebeam & Shinkfield, 2007). Accuracy includes standards that require evaluators to describe the program as it was planned and executed, present the program background and setting, collect and convey technically accurate information, and report valid and reliable findings (CDC, 1999; Saewert, 2013). The accuracy standards focus on justified conclusions and decisions, valid and reliable information, clear descriptions of the program and context, systematic information management, sound designs and analyses, explicit evaluation reasoning, and effective communication and reporting (Yarbrough, Shulha, Hopson, & Caruthers, 2011).

Evaluation Accountability

A new attribute, *evaluation accountability*, refers to the adequate documentation of processes, agreements, data files and reports, and an internal and external perspective focused on improvement and accountability of processes and products (Ruhe & Boudreau, 2013). Even evaluations need to be evaluated. Quality improvement is an ongoing process, but events that lead to quality improvement efforts need to be reviewed as well (Haleem et al., 2010). The evaluation accountability standards encourage adequate documentation of the evaluation and an internal and external review of the evaluation, also known as meta-evaluation (Yarbrough, Shulha, Hopson, & Caruthers, 2011).

FRAMEWORK FOR EVALUATION: IDEAL OR OPTIMAL?

Nursing programs cannot question *whether* to evaluate their work, but instead, *how*. What is the best way to evaluate? What are we learning from the evaluation? How will we use the learning to make programs more effective and accountable? The challenge is to devise an optimal—as opposed to an ideal—strategy. An optimal strategy is one that accomplishes each step in a framework in a way that accommodates the program context and meets or exceeds all relevant standards (CDC, 1999). With numerous models and theories to guide evaluation, selection of an evaluation model depends on the needs of the stakeholders who will use the evaluation results (Hackbarth & Gall, 2005). With no clear consensus or agreement about the use of any one model in program evaluation, and with various frameworks and methods employed, any of the models can be used to: analyze new or existing programs; produce information for evaluating the program's effectiveness; and use this information to make decisions about program refinement, revisions, and/or continuation (Saewert, 2013).

Sohn (1987) asserted that, although models provide a philosophical and procedural framework, and some guidelines for evaluation generally help people conduct an evaluation, they may be of little value in telling evaluators *what* to do and should not dictate the actual evaluation *process*. Consequently, thoughtful consideration is needed to make a theoretical model practical, functional, and adaptable to a program's context and to avoid rigid adherence to a particular model.

Although theoretically possible, a perfect evaluation plan is rare (Hammer & Bentley, 2003). Table 2.2 presents an overview of eight selected models for program evaluation: objective-based, goal-free, expert-oriented, naturalistic, participative-oriented, improvement-focused, success case, and theory-driven. Considerations for the use of each model accompany the description. Existing models are used in a complementary manner or as a foundation for developing new evaluation strategies (Stavropoulou & Stroubouki, 2014).

TABLE 2.2

Overview of Selected Models for Program Evaluation

Model	Description	Considerations
Objective-based	Uses objectives written by the creators of the program and evaluator. Objectives depict the overarching purpose of the evaluation and guide the type of information to be used in the evaluation. With this approach, the evaluation is based on stated program goals and objectives. Evaluation data collection activities stem from the objectives.	Most prevalent model used for program evaluation. Some evaluators become so focused on the objectives that they neglect to examine why programs succeed or fail, consider any additional positive or undesired effects of the program, or ask whether the program objectives were the best ones to represent program stakeholder interests and requirements.
Goal-free	Assumption is that evaluators work more effectively if they do not know the goals of the program. Considerable time is spent studying the program as administered, stakeholders, and setting, and recording documentation to identify program impacts.	Approach is expensive, rather open-ended, and may be experienced as threatening. Programs are required to show specific outcomes. If outcomes are not included in the evaluation, the appropriate data may not be collected.

TABLE 2.2

Overview of Selected Models for Program Evaluation *(Continued)*

Model	Description	Considerations
Expert-oriented	Focus is on the evaluator as a content expert who carefully examines the program to render judgment about its quality. Evaluators judge a program on the basis of an established set of criteria as well as their own expertise in the area. Some decisions are based on objective quantified information as well as on qualitative impressions. This approach is often used when the program being evaluated is large, complex, and unique.	Agencies that grant accreditation to institutions, program, or services send program evaluators to conduct an on-site, expert-oriented evaluation. Examples include relevant accrediting and licensing bodies and agencies. Issues include specificity of criteria, interpretation of criteria by experts, and level of the evaluator's content expertise.
Naturalistic	Used to develop a deep and thorough understanding of the program. Evaluator becomes the data gatherer, using a variety of observation and qualitative techniques. By personally observing all phases of the program and holding detailed conversations with key stakeholders, the evaluator attempts to gain a rich understanding of the program, stakeholder interests, and the environment and setting.	Because of the detail included, reports often become lengthy. Personal observations may serve as an advantage to understand the meaning of numerical information about the program.
Participative-oriented	Evaluators seek to involve program participants in evaluation of the program. Evaluators invite stakeholders to actively participate in evaluation while gaining skills from the experience. Participants may develop instruments, analyze data, and report findings.	Requires close contact with stakeholders. Some argue that this approach can compromise validity of the evaluation. Potential benefits include: stakeholders may be more likely to enact recommendations and the process for improvement may take less time.

(continued)

TABLE 2.2

Overview of Selected Models for Program Evaluation *(Continued)*

Model	Description	Considerations
Improvement-focused	Evaluators adopt an explicit assumption that program improvement is the focus of the evaluation. Evaluators help the program discover discrepancies between: the program objectives and the needs of the target population, program implementation and plans, and the expectations of the target population and program delivered.	Approach tends to lead to an integrated understanding of the program and its effects. Some experts believe that an improvement-focused approach best meets the criteria necessary for effective evaluation. Approach may be experienced as threatening.
Success case	Detailed information is sought from those who benefit most from the program.	Approach could lead to tailoring a program to those who benefit most from the program to the exclusion of other key stakeholder interests and needs.
Theory-driven	Evaluations are based on a description of the program offered, the way the program is expected to change the participants, and specific outcomes to be achieved. Analysis consists of discovering the relationships among: program services and the characteristics of the participants, program services and immediate changes, and immediate changes and outcome variables.	Complex correlation techniques are used to analyze data and relationships. Qualitative understanding of the program may be ignored in place of quantitative approaches. May require resources and expertise that are not available.

Adapted from: Saewert, K. J. (2013). Program evaluation. In M. A. Mateo & M. D. Foreman (Eds.), *Research for advanced practice nurses: From evidence to practice* (2nd ed., pp. 283–319). New York: Springer. Reprinted with permission.

The CDC framework for program evaluations, illustrated in Figure 2.1, is a practical, nonprescriptive tool, designed to summarize and organize the essential elements of program evaluation. It includes recommended steps in evaluation and standards for effective evaluation, and is a starting point for tailoring a program evaluation (Saewert, 2013). This framework was developed specifically to be a resource for people to plan and carry out a comprehensive review of their own evaluation activities and outcomes, communicate

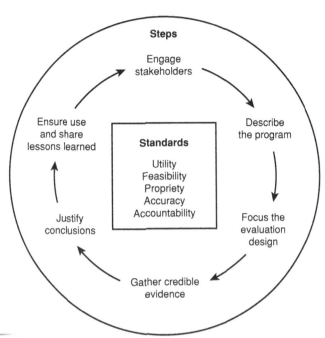

FIGURE 2.1 Framework for program evaluation. Adapted from: Saewert, K. J. (2013). Program evaluation. In M. A. Mateo & M. D. Foreman (Eds.), *Research for advanced practice nurses: From evidence to practice* (2nd ed., pp. 283–319). New York: Springer. Reprinted with permission. Originally adapted from the Centers for Disease Control and Prevention (http://www.cdc.gov/eval/framework).

priorities about evaluation, train staff members, and engage the community (Milstein & Wetterhall, 2000). Ultimately, the selection of an evaluation model should consider the needs of the stakeholders who will use the evaluation results. Evaluators should look for a model that will help organize the evaluation and yield the most useful information for various stakeholders (Hackbarth & Gall, 2005). It is conceivable to use an eclectic approach in which members of a nursing program do not select any particular model but design their own by purposeful selection of pertinent aspects from more than one model (Sohn, 1987).

Stavropoulou and Stroubouki (2014) asserted that following a certain model restricts experimentation and discovery in the modern era of evaluation. Instead, synthesis of methods and approaches can be transformative. Evaluators should recognize that:

1. models and specific approaches in evaluation can assist faculty, administrators, and other evaluators by providing alternatives, ideas, and concepts that help to formulate the appropriate evaluation strategy for the school's unique investigation;

2. synthesis of evaluation models is not only possible but also evident most of the time, because program evaluation is seldom guided by a specific evaluation model; and,

3. models and methods of evaluation are a representation of the imperfect real world of evaluation and, as such, should be viewed with caution.

A focus on minimum standards is no longer acceptable for programs striving to attract and retain outstanding students and faculty and to prepare graduates who can provide the leadership needed for increasingly complex health care environments (Valiga, 2003). Nursing licensure boards and accreditation bodies expect curricula to be ever changing and dynamic. Accordingly, a dynamic nursing curriculum is relevant and ever changing. It should be evaluated for rigor as well as to determine if it is meaningful and relevant to all stakeholders, including students, faculty, and the community (Pross, 2010).

Finally, optimizing program evaluation in modern educational contexts requires individuals who *engage* in an organizational culture that *supports* evaluation. Requisite individual and organizational attributes include: openness, commitment, expertise, readiness to change, self-confidence, teamwork, administrative support, infrastructure, resources, experimentation, willingness to fail, vision, and optimism (Stavropoulou & Stroubouki, 2014).

SUMMARY

Program evaluation presents an opportunity to engage in a process that can be leveraged as a catalyst for change and program improvement. It is a means by which nurse educators can gain a better understanding of what we do and the effects of our actions. Nurse educators evaluate, among many components, their approaches to teaching, course and curricular outcomes, student learning, faculty productivity, and clinical expertise and performance. It follows that we would apply these same practices to the educational programs in which we teach.

The process of evaluation should lead to the use of findings by a variety of stakeholders. The importance of using what is learned from program evaluation is critical. For this to occur, program evaluation must be understandable, relevant, meaningful, credible, and focused on actions or decisions leading to program- and organization-level learning and improvement. Optimal program evaluation is accomplished through assigning value to evaluation, making sound evaluative judgments, putting evaluation principles into practice, and meeting evaluation standards.

References

American Evaluation Association. (2004). American Evaluation Association Guiding Principles for Evaluators. Retrieved from http://www.eval.org/p/cm/ld/fid=51.

Billings, J. R. (2000). Community development: A critical review of approaches to evaluation. *Journal of Advanced Nursing, 31*, 472–480. doi:10.1046/j.1365-2648.2000.01278.x

Centers for Disease Control and Prevention. (1999). Framework for program evaluation in public health. *Morbidity and Mortality Weekly Report (MMWR) 48*(No. RR-11), 1–42.

Hackbarth, D., & Gall, G. B. (2005). Evaluation of school-based health center programs and services: The whys and hows of demonstrating program effectiveness. *Nursing Clinics of North America, 40*, 711–724. doi: 10.1016/j.cnur.2005.07.008

Haleem, D. M., Evanina, K., Gallagher, R., Golden, M. A., Healy-Karabell, K., & Manetti, W. (2010). Program evaluation: How faculty addressed concerns about the nursing program. *Nurse Educator, 35,* 118–121. doi:10.1097/NNE.0b013e3181d95000

Hammer, J. B., & Bently, R. W. (2003). A systematic evaluation plan that works. *Nurse Educator, 28,* 179–184.

Lewallen, L. P. (2015). Practical strategies for nursing education program evaluation. *Journal of Professional Nursing, 31,* 133–140. doi:10.1016/j.profnurs.2014.09.002

Milstein, B., & Wetterhall, S. (2000). A framework featuring steps and standards for program evaluation. *Health Promotion Practice, 1,* 221–228.

Posavac, E. J., & Carey, R. G. (2010). *Program evaluation: Methods and case studies* (8th ed.). Upper Saddle River, NJ: Pearson Education.

Pross, E. A. (2010). Promoting excellence in nursing education (PENE): Pross evaluation model. *Nurse Education Today, 30,* 557–561. doi:10.1016/j.nedt.2009.11.010

Ruhe, V., & Boudreau, J. D. (2013). The 2011 program evaluation standards: A framework for quality in medical education programmes. *Journal of Evaluation in Clinical Practice, 19,* 925–932. doi:10.1111/j.1365-2753.2012.01879.x

Saewert, K. J. (2013). Program evaluation. In M. A. Mateo & M. D. Foreman (Eds.), *Research for advanced practice nurses: From evidence to practice* (2nd ed., pp. 283–319). New York: Springer.

Sarnecky, M. T. (1990). Program evaluation part 1: Four generations of theory. *Nurse Educator, 15*(5), 25–28.

Shadish, W. R., Jr., Cook, T. D., & Leviton, L. C. (1991). *Foundations of program evaluation: Theories of practice.* Thousand Oaks, CA: Sage.

Sohn, K. S. (1987). Program evaluation in nursing. *Nurse Educator, 12*(2), 27–34.

Spaulding, D. T. (2008). *Program evaluation in practice: Core concepts and examples for discussion and analysis.* San Francisco, CA: Jossey-Bass.

Stavropoulou, A., & Stroubouki, T. (2014). Evaluation of educational programs: The contribution of history to modern evaluation thinking. *Health Science Journal, 8,* 193–204.

Stufflebeam, D. L., & Shinkfield, A. J. (2007). *Evaluation theory, models and applications.* San Francisco, CA: Jossey-Bass.

Valiga, T. (2003). The pursuit of excellence in nursing education. *Nursing Education Perspectives, 24,* 275–277.

Yarbrough, D. B., Shulha, L. M., Hopson, R. K., & Caruthers, F. A. (2011). *The program evaluation standards: A guide for evaluations and evaluation users* (3rd ed.). Thousand Oaks, CA: Sage.

3

Curriculum Evaluation

Theresa M. "Terry" Valiga, EdD, RN, CNE, FAAN, ANEF

Faculty in schools of nursing often spend a great deal of time designing a curriculum that provides students with an organized approach to learning their new nursing role, implementing that curriculum in ways that engage the learner and effectively employ creative strategies, and evaluating what students have learned as a result of those experiences. However, efforts to evaluate the entire curriculum are often overlooked, are not approached in a systematic way, and are incomplete. This chapter addresses the purposes of and ways to approach curriculum evaluation and relate this activity to the overall program evaluation. In addition, this chapter clarifies the role of faculty in the curriculum development, evaluation, and revision process.

CURRICULUM DEVELOPMENT AND EVALUATION

Often, when we think of *curriculum,* we think of a collection of courses, the rigid sequencing of courses, the content to be covered, the required prerequisites, credit allocation, the ratio between credits and hours, and even the plan to achieve desired licensing or certification examination results. But a curriculum is much more than these things. In essence, the curriculum is a *gestalt* that incorporates hoped-for, as well as unanticipated, outcomes; the variety of experiences designed to enhance student learning; the assessment and evaluation methods used; the diverse pedagogical perspectives of faculty; and the relationships between and among students and teachers. It also has been referred to as stories to be heard (Ironside, 2004; Tanner, 2004); a culture of excellence; the full engagement of participants in learning and growing; and the complex and dynamic interactions among students, teachers, learning experiences, the material to be learned, and the values to be reflected upon.

Therefore, when evaluating a curriculum, it is not enough to focus only on student evaluations of courses or teachers, peer review of a teaching session or an online course, graduation rates, or licensure or certification examination pass rates. All components of the curriculum need to be examined for the extent to which they are relevant, effective, and critical to developing graduates who can thrive in today's uncertain, ambiguous, technology-rich, ever-changing health care environment, and who can shape the future of health care and the nursing profession.

CURRICULUM EVALUATION AND PROGRAM EVALUATION

Program evaluation addresses all of the elements needed to offer a quality nursing program and prepare graduates for practice roles. The *Excellence in Nursing Education Model* of the National League for Nursing (NLN, 2006) provides an overview of these components: well-prepared faculty; qualified students; well-prepared educational administrators; clear program standards and hallmarks that raise expectations; recognition of expertise; quality and adequate resources; evidence-based program and teaching and evaluation methods; and student-centered, interactive, innovative programs and curricula.

Thus, ongoing evaluation of an overall program requires a careful look at many elements, one of which is the curriculum. It is clear that, to implement the curriculum, well-prepared faculty are needed, as are administrative support and resources that are adequate and of high quality. Therefore, curriculum evaluation cannot be complete unless many of these components are addressed; however, program evaluation is a larger concept that subsumes curriculum evaluation.

CURRICULUM COMPONENTS TO EVALUATE

What are the essential components that need to be studied to determine the relevance and effectiveness of the curriculum? They begin with the school's philosophy and end with the detailed resources needed to facilitate and assess student learning.

Philosophy

The school's philosophy is an expression of the values and beliefs of the faculty regarding human beings, health, health care, the environment or context, nurses and nursing practice, and teaching/learning. It is important that faculty regularly review the school's philosophy and reflect on whether the beliefs expressed in it remain current and the extent to which the expressed beliefs and values truly guide day-to-day actions. For example, the philosophy may indicate that the faculty support individualized, student-centered learning. On reflection, however, faculty may realize that there is little or no opportunity throughout the curriculum for students to follow their individualized passions, learn in ways that are most effective for them, or do anything other than follow the teacher-directed path. Such a realization would hopefully lead faculty to reflect on how deeply this value is held and what they may need to do differently to "make it come alive" and be more than mere words on a page. Since values and beliefs are not expected to change dramatically in a short period of time, it is not necessary to engage in deep reflection about the philosophy every semester or on an annual basis; this might be an activity that is undertaken with seriousness every 5 to 6 years.

Conceptual Framework

Although most schools do not use a single theory—nursing or otherwise—as the framework for the curriculum, there needs to be some type of "umbrella" that guides faculty in writing program outcomes, designing the learning sequence, and deciding where to place emphases. The concepts may be pervasive (i.e., consistently addressed regardless of where students are in the program), or they may be progressive in nature (i.e., developed in increasing depth and complexity from the beginning to the end of the program). Regardless of the nature of a particular concept, it is essential that the key concepts that undergird the entire curriculum be relevant, clearly defined, and understood by all. Again, the concepts that serve as the framework for the curriculum are not likely to change often, but it is essential that faculty regularly reflect on whether they are congruent with current discussions about health, health care, and nursing practice. As a result of ongoing environmental scanning and literature review, it becomes increasingly clear that today's nursing curricula must help students develop the understanding, skills, and values needed to engage effectively in collaborative practice that is based on evidence.

Program Outcomes

Program outcomes are statements of student achievement, specifying what they should know, be able to do, and value or appreciate upon completion of the program. They are important because they allow for accountability, serve as a basis for evaluation of the effectiveness of the program, are essential for accreditation requirements, clarify what employers should expect, and give direction to future program planning.

Since the most central indication of academic quality is student learning, program outcomes must be *student-focused*. Additionally, because they reflect the totality of student achievement as the result of the entire course of study, program outcomes should be *complex* and *multifaceted*.

When evaluating program outcomes, faculty should consider the clarity with which they have defined the qualities and characteristics of graduates on completion of the program, the realities of today's practice arenas, whether they address preparing graduates for an unknown future and a lifetime career, the values expressed in the school's philosophy, the concepts articulated in the framework, and new insights about learning. Consideration also should be given to characteristics of the school's unique student body, time available to realistically achieve the outcome, and resources available to achieve the stated ends. Finally, program outcomes should use unambiguous language and be measurable. However, it is important to remember that multiple means to measure achievement of the outcomes is essential in light of their complexity and multi-faceted nature.

Level Outcomes

Level outcomes can be thought of as the "signposts" along the journey to the overall program outcomes. A school may define a "level" in any number of ways, for example, by academic year or by semester, but it is important to remember that the "cluster" of courses included in a level should have some consistency among them. For example, a school may define Level I as the first semester of the program, where the focus is on laying a foundation related to the profession of nursing, basic knowledge and skills, and wellness. Level II might include semesters two, three, and four, in which the focus is on caring for different patient populations (e.g., children, pregnant women, and the elderly) and the nursing care needed to help them maintain or regain health. Finally, Level III might include the final two semesters of the program, which focus on caring for complex patient situations, collaborating with the interprofessional team, functioning as a leader, and making the transition from the role of student to that of graduate nurse.

Level outcomes, then, should define the expected accomplishments of students as a result of the learning experiences in all courses in that level; thus, they complement, but are different from, individual course objectives. Additionally, they should show increasing complexity of student knowledge, skills, and values as the student moves from one level to the next.

When evaluating a program's level outcomes, faculty should look for clarity, congruence with the program outcomes, and whether the outcomes are realistic, given the course experiences included in a particular level. If there is a mismatch between course experiences and level outcomes, faculty need to decide if the courses are not designed well enough to help students achieve the level outcomes or if level outcomes are unrealistic. Faculty also should examine whether the level outcomes truly progress in complexity and serve to illustrate the unique focus of each level, how each level builds on the previous one, and whether all are leading toward accomplishment of the program outcomes.

Curriculum Design

The curriculum design is the sequence in which students take courses: in nursing; in foundational physical, social, and behavioral sciences; in the liberal arts; and electives. To evaluate the design, faculty need to assess the extent to which students have the necessary foundation, what students have learned in foundational or prerequisite courses on which to build nursing courses (Valiga, 2015); degree of flexibility in the course of study; logical flow of course experiences; extent to which the values expressed in the philosophy and concepts articulated in the framework are evident; and extent to which the "collection" of courses in any given semester are aligned with the level—and ultimately, program—outcomes.

Courses

Evaluation of courses is often done only through the use of student feedback on end-of-term standardized forms. While such an approach is valuable, it is not sufficient.

Course evaluations also should address whether students came into the course with the necessary foundation, the degree to which faculty repeated foundational knowledge, the depth of student learning, and the extent to which students and faculty believe that the foundation needed to be successful in subsequent courses has been built. Additionally, courses should be evaluated in terms of the effectiveness of methods used in the course (e.g., case studies, team-based learning, textbooks) in facilitating learning, and the appropriateness of assessment and evaluation methods used in the course to judge student attainment of the objectives. Finally, consideration should be given to the nature of the learning environment that existed in the course, ways in which student-student and student-teacher interactions were encouraged, and the degree to which the learning needs of the diverse student population were met.

Teaching/Learning Strategies

The primary considerations that must be given when evaluating the teaching and learning strategies used in a course are whether they effectively facilitated student learning and the degree to which they engaged students as active learners. Faculty also should ensure that the strategies used were based in evidence—not tradition—and were designed and implemented in accord with best practices.

Whether students liked using case studies, brainstorming, or concept maps is helpful to know, but the more important question addresses the extent to which those approaches helped students learn. Additionally, while it is important to know if faculty liked teaching online or using gaming as a strategy, it is critical to determine if the course was well organized, made reasonable expectations of students, ensured that students were adequately prepared to engage in specific learning activities, and was implemented effectively.

Assessment/Evaluation Methods

Similar to evaluating teaching/learning strategies, faculty need to evaluate the effectiveness of the methods used in the course to determine student achievement of the course objectives. Questions should be raised about the fairness of methods, reasonableness of how each is weighted when calculating the course grade, the variety of approaches used, and the rationale for each method. In addition, faculty should ensure that each of the domains of learning appropriate to the course—cognitive, psychomotor, and affective—are assessed. For example, if only multiple-choice tests are used to assess student learning, does that convey a message to students that only cognitive knowing is important?

Assessment/evaluation methods also should focus on students' writing, speaking, presentation, and leadership skills; their ability to manage uncertainty and ambiguity; the effectiveness of their interactions with others (patients, classmates, nurses in clinical settings, and members of the health care team); the clarity and strength of their own values; and an understanding of how personal values influence their behaviors. Faculty may find that there is a need to identify some courses as writing-intensive so that students are challenged to develop those skills throughout the program. Or they may determine that certain courses should include professional presentations for students to get feedback on their ability to present in an organized fashion, argue convincingly, respond to questions from others, "think on their feet," and speak in an articulate manner. Thus, evaluation of assessment/evaluation methods involves more than merely doing item analyses on a multiple-choice test to determine if a question is a good one or not.

Resources and Partnerships

The final curriculum component to be evaluated relates to the resources available to support course implementation and student achievement of course objectives, and ultimately level and program outcomes. Such resources include physical space, user-friendliness of online learning management systems, laboratory equipment and supplies, library resources, clinical facilities, counseling resources, writing skills resources, and faculty qualifications and teaching abilities. It also is important to reflect on the nature of partnerships that have been established in various inpatient clinical units, outpatient clinics, home care agencies, community agencies, and others. A "breakdown" in any of these areas can sorely undermine the effectiveness of a curriculum; thus, they must be attended to carefully and seriously as the curriculum is evaluated.

STANDARDS AND INDICATORS

One might wonder about the standards to use when evaluating a curriculum and all its component parts. Two key resources for standards are accreditation criteria used by the NLN Commission for Nursing Education Accreditation (2015) and the American Association of Colleges of Nursing Commission on Collegiate Nursing Education (2015). Other resources include the outcomes and competencies for graduates of all types of nursing programs (NLN, 2010) and the NLN's *Hallmarks of Excellence in Nursing Education* (2015). Each of these resources provides ideas or standards related to curriculum development, implementation, and impact, and each is an excellent source for faculty as they engage in curriculum evaluation activities.

Unlike accreditation standards, which set minimum standards for quality academic programs, the NLN's *Hallmarks of Excellence* (2015) outline a level of achievement that exceeds the minimum and challenges faculty to use even higher standards to design and evaluate their programs. In the Curriculum section of that document, the following are examples of stated hallmarks (NLN, 2015):

- The curriculum provides experiential cultural learning activities that enhance students' abilities to think critically, reflect thoughtfully, and provide culturally sensitive, evidence-based nursing care to diverse populations.
- The curriculum emphasizes students' values development, socialization to the new role, commitment to lifelong learning, and creativity.
- The curriculum is evidence-based.

Using these hallmarks, and the indicators outlined for each, challenges faculty to think deeply about what they are trying to accomplish through their curriculum and serves as a basis for curriculum evaluation. Whatever the standards or indicators used, faculty should "set the bar high" and not settle for mediocrity. The preparation of graduates for the significant roles that they will have in the future requires that faculty strive for excellence and not be satisfied with the status quo or merely doing things the way that they have always been done.

DATA COLLECTION STRATEGIES

As mentioned earlier, the primary sources of data about the effectiveness of the curriculum often include only student evaluations of courses and teachers, along with pass rates on licensing or certification examinations. There is no question that such measures are important, but they are not sufficient. Instead, data should be collected from many stakeholders, using varied strategies to obtain a comprehensive view of how well the curriculum is doing what faculty hoped that it would do.

There is no one-and-only-one or one "right" way to collect data about the effectiveness of the curriculum. Therefore, faculty have the freedom to construct approaches that are workable for them and that will yield information to help them determine what to continue, what to modify, what to change dramatically, what to eliminate, and when a major curriculum revision is needed. Examples of options for data collection about the curriculum include:

- **Plan annual retreats** that focus on a "deep dive" into all or part of the curriculum. For example, one year, the focus might be on the constellation of courses in Level I, in which faculty look critically at the degree to which those courses are congruent with the school's philosophy and framework, the extent to which they align with the level outcomes, what faculty teaching in subsequent courses say about the preparedness of students as they enter those upper-level courses, the effectiveness of any writing-intensive courses, the variety of teaching and learning strategies and assessment/ evaluation methods used, what students said about their experiences, feedback from clinical staff who worked with students, student performance on tests and other measures of their learning, and so on. This 360-degree review of Level I would lead faculty to make recommendations about any changes that might be needed and what they would look for to determine if those changes were effective. In the following year, the same process could be applied to the constellation of courses in Level II, and so forth, until data are collected on each level of the curriculum.

- **Use the Self-Assessment Checklist** developed by Adams and Valiga (2009, pp. 163-179) and based on the *Hallmarks of Excellence in Nursing Education* (NLN, 2015). Faculty might be asked to complete the checklist individually, then—again in a retreat-like forum— compare their responses, discuss areas with widely divergent views, and determine what changes, if any, are needed to meet the hallmarks.

- **Invite an external curriculum expert** (from another part of the university or from another school) to review the curriculum, examining internal consistency among all the components and how the curriculum aligns with selected accreditation standards or other benchmarks. This individual could then engage in dialogue with faculty about areas of strength and concern, and how those areas of concern could be addressed.

- **Conduct focus groups or open dialogue** with clinical partners on a regular basis. Faculty should seek input on how graduates of their nursing program compare to graduates of other programs in terms of their ability to think critically, provide quality care, work collaboratively with others, and meet other expectations. This also would be an excellent opportunity to discuss the quality of students' clinical experiences, supportiveness of clinical staff, extent to which students and clinical instructors perceive that they are an integral part of the practice environment, communication patterns, and other elements that impact the quality and effectiveness of student clinical experiences.

- **Critically reflect on the philosophy** to determine if the values expressed in it still reflect the thinking of the faculty. As mentioned, this might be done only every 5 to 6 years, but it is a step that should not be forgotten. One way to approach this analysis is to create a survey that asks faculty to examine each sentence in the philosophy and provide input on whether they think it continues to be accurate and essential, is important but does not need to be stated in the philosophy, is no longer congruent with current practice or trends, and so forth. Faculty also could be asked to share values that may be absent from the current document and should be added. A team could do an analysis of the survey results, share them with the faculty as a whole or in smaller groups, discuss the findings, and make recommendations for changes that might be needed in the document.

- **Critically reflect on the framework** to determine if the key concepts on which the curriculum has been built remain relevant and if all concepts essential for contemporary nursing practice (e.g., interprofessional collaboration, evidence-based practice, patient-centered care, information management) are incorporated and fully developed. Such an analysis would be enhanced by careful environmental scanning, in which faculty have reviewed the essence of key documents, organizational recommendations, current literature, and input from stakeholders such as alumni and employers. The key points from these resources could be summarized and "plotted against" the existing curriculum concepts to identify areas of congruence and where the curriculum concepts might be deficient or paying inadequate attention considering today's environment and the yet-to-be-determined environment of the future.

WHAT DO THE DATA MEAN?

Once faculty have engaged in activities such as the ones suggested earlier, as well as those described in Chapter 6 and other chapters in this book, they are then challenged to reflect on what those data mean and the implications for curriculum refinement or revision, or major "overhaul." During this phase of curriculum development, faculty need to be willing to abandon "sacred cows" and to accept that courses they have been teaching may need significant revision in terms of the objectives and focus, teaching/learning strategies, and/or evaluation methods.

Faculty may discover that the values expressed in the philosophy are not really guiding the design or implementation of the curriculum, or they may unearth many disconnects among the various curriculum components. For example, concepts identified in the framework may be evident only in beginning courses but not integrated throughout the program, or concepts may be emphasized in final-semester courses that have not even been introduced previously. They may find that the curriculum is not effective in helping students develop their identities as nurses, nurse practitioners, or scholars. Interpreting the meaning of curriculum evaluation data also may highlight for faculty that they cannot understand the data because they have not established benchmarks for what they expect to achieve.

Although it is possible that data from curriculum evaluation efforts reveal that everything is perfect and no revisions are needed, the greater likelihood is that a number of areas needing attention will be identified. Faculty then need to weigh the significance of each area and its impact on preparing students effectively, and outline plans for which areas to address as a priority, which are not urgent, and which could be improved but also could remain unchanged. Such discussions are likely to reveal faculty beliefs and values about nursing practice, educational approaches, and student-teacher relationships, all of which provide an excellent opportunity to go back to the philosophy.

The goal of a curriculum is not to make everyone happy, as that is impossible. However, if the most significant guiding principles are "What is best for student learning?" and "What will help us best prepare students for today's and tomorrow's world?," consensus can be reached and appropriate curriculum refinements or revisions can be made.

SUMMARY

In conclusion, it is important to remember that curriculum evaluation is an ongoing and complex process that must involve all faculty. Input must be sought from all stakeholders—students, faculty, clinical partners, employers, administrators—to obtain a comprehensive view of what is effective and what needs improvement. Additionally, it is critical to keep in mind that a change in one component of the curriculum will impact other components. The curriculum must be conceptualized as a gestalt, and attention must be paid to the complex and dynamic interactions among students, teachers, learning experiences, the material to be learned, and the values to be reflected upon.

Curriculum revisions should be implemented thoughtfully, and faculty should be sensitive to avoid allowing existing practices to become "carved in stone." Instead, a curriculum should be thought of as a living, dynamic entity that evolves along with the needs of society, the nursing profession, and individual schools. Nursing students and the patients, families, and communities for whom they will care deserve nothing less.

References

Adams, M. H., & Valiga, T. M. (2009). *Achieving excellence in nursing education*. New York, NY: National League for Nursing.

American Association of Colleges of Nursing. (2015). *Standards, procedures and resources*. Retrieved from http://www.aacn.nche.edu/ccne-accreditation/standards-procedures-resources/overview.

Ironside, P. M. (2004). "Covering content" and teaching thinking: Deconstructing the additive curriculum. *Journal of Nursing Education, 43*(1), 5–12.

National League for Nursing. (2006). *Excellence in nursing education model*. Retrieved from http://www.nln.org/professional-development-programs/teaching-resources/excellence-model.

National League for Nursing. (2010). *Outcomes and competencies for graduates of practical/vocational, diploma, associate degree, baccalaureate, master's practice doctorate, and research doctorate programs in nursing*. New York, NY: Author.

National League for Nursing. (2015). *Hallmarks of excellence in nursing education*.

Retrieved from http://www.nln.org/profes-
sional-development-programs/teaching-
resources/hallmarks-of-excellence.

National League for Nursing Commission
for Nursing Education Accreditation.
(2015). *Proposed standards for accreditation*. Retrieved from http://www.nln.org/
accreditation-services/proposed-standards-
for-accreditation.

Tanner, C. A. (2004). The meaning of curriculum: Content to be covered or stories
to be heard? *Journal of Nursing Education,
43*(1), 3–4.

Valiga, T. M. (2015). Rethinking prerequisites.
Journal of Nursing Education, 54, 183–184.
doi: 10.3928/01484834-20150318-10.

4

Formulating Evaluation Questions

Thomas Christenbery, PhD, RN, CNE

Many published, well-established questionnaires measure phenomena central to nursing education such as critical thinking (Facione & Facione, 2008) and self-efficacy (Stump, Husman, & Brem, 2012). However, none of these are generally accepted questionnaires measuring program outcomes or stakeholder satisfaction related to school of nursing program evaluation. When evaluating schools of nursing, faculty and program evaluators often construct their own program-specific survey or questionnaires. Schools of nursing use questionnaires as a primary tool for generating information that is analyzed to provide important decision points regarding both program outcomes and stakeholder satisfaction. The purpose of this chapter is to provide guidelines for (1) writing survey questions, (2) selecting questions to plan evaluation, (3) identifying appropriate indicators for questions, and (4) planning data collection for school of nursing program evaluation.

THE POWER OF THE PROGRAM EVALUATION QUESTION

Voltaire's maxim that people should be judged by their questions rather than by their answers applies to program evaluation questions (BookBrowse, 2015). Good evaluation questions produce critical information, prompt important concerns from key stakeholders, help distinguish what parts of a program are working or not working, and thus identify how future program aspects may be improved (Fitzpatrick, Sanders, & Worthen, 2011). Before developing and selecting evaluation questions, wise evaluators carefully analyze the nursing program's mission and objectives to create questions that will specifically address how best to influence the program and its outcomes (Cizek, 2010). Importantly, the choice of questions defines what a nursing program may need to change for enhancement of quality nursing education. Carefully created and selected evaluation questions reflect a nursing program's current goals and determine future program goals.

Well-developed survey questions are essential components of a successful program evaluation process. Questions that accurately assess the nursing program and its stakeholders' attributes and concerns are critical for optimal program evaluation (Dillman, Smyth, & Christian, 2014). Appropriate sampling and high response rates are insufficient for providing desired survey results if data gathered were derived from ambiguous or biased questions (Pew Research Center, 2015). Question development is a multi-stage process requiring team-focused attention to question development and selection. The question development and selection process is challenging as questions can cover topics in varying degrees of detail, can be asked in multiple ways, and if asked earlier in a survey can have a high probability of influencing how participants respond to later questions.

IDENTIFYING THE PURPOSE OF THE SURVEY

Generally, surveys or questionnaires are one of the most effective means for collecting program evaluation data (Fitzpatrick et al., 2011; Rossi, Lipsey, & Freeman, 2004). Several activities are helpful in clarifying the purpose of the survey and thus instructive for question development. First, evaluators need to determine what they intend to learn from the survey. A clear understanding of the survey's purpose aids in identifying the type of information to be collected. To illustrate, evaluators need to consider if the primary purpose of the survey is to evaluate program *outcomes,* stakeholder *satisfaction,* or a combination of both outcomes and satisfaction. Outcomes are concerned with determining whether a particular intervention contributed to producing a particular result. For example, does the school's National Council Licensure Examination (NCLEX®) review course affect first-time pass rates for graduates? Satisfaction is concerned with what effect a particular aspect of the program may have on the quality of life of stakeholders. For instance, do web-based chats in distance courses enhance students' perception of belonging?

Second, evaluators need to consider who will be evaluated. Identifying the target participants assists evaluators in deciding what type of data to collect from the participants (Fitzpatrick et al., 2011). For example, evaluators may be interested in better understanding the perceived level of confidence that graduates have in performing health assessments at the completion of the program. If the program has multiple exit points, such as Bachelor of Science in Nursing (BSN) and Master of Science in Nursing (MSN), questions need to be tailored to the academic and skill level of each group of potential respondents.

Third, evaluators need to consider who will be the primary recipients receiving the report and how recipients will use the report's findings. Understanding the evaluation needs of a specific recipient group supports the process of developing targeted questions to address those needs. Scholarly productivity of alumni is a critical program outcome in which both faculty and school of nursing administrators are keenly interested. If the recipients of an alumni productivity survey are faculty, questions may need to focus on evaluating *academic activities* that enhance future productivity. If the alumni productivity survey recipients are administrators, questions may need to be targeted to evaluate the merit of *specific school resources* that fostered scholarly productivity. A clear understanding of the survey's purpose, who will be evaluated, and who will receive the survey's results for utilization are essential for evaluators to know before writing and selecting evaluation questions.

CHARACTERISTICS OF A GOOD EVALUATION QUESTION

Meaningful program evaluation results are dependent upon well-thought-out, relevant evaluation questions. Evaluation questions are often born from information that accreditation agencies and key internal and external stakeholders need to know about nursing programs. Information requested from accreditation agencies (e.g., National League for Nursing Commission for Nursing Education Accreditation, Accreditation Agency for Midwifery) and key stakeholders (e.g., faculty, alumni, students) is copious, often complex, and highly varied. It is a daunting task to determine what questions will provide all interested agencies and stakeholders the critical information that they request (Stufflebeam & Shinkfield, 2007). Poorly worded questions are confusing and can cause respondents to provide erroneous data that are useless to the school's program evaluation process. Therefore, the evaluation team needs a clear understanding of how to create and select evaluation questions that provide maximum and accurate information with optimal efficiency. To begin the process of optimal question development, it is essential for the evaluation team to identify the purpose for conducting the survey.

Types of Evaluation Questions

Numerous types of questions may be considered for an evaluation. To give structure to an evaluation, it is helpful to classify the types of questions into one of three categories that provide methodological support for question development and selection. Evaluation questions acquire formation when classified as descriptive, normative, or outcome/impact (Mertens, 2010).

Descriptive questions provide a depiction of the nursing program as both an entity and process (Stufflebeam & Shinkfield, 2007). In general, program evaluation surveys include descriptive questions that seek to identify and define program characteristics, stakeholder perceptions, and organizational relationships. Asking graduates, in an exit survey, to rate the school's financial aid services is an example of a descriptive question. Descriptive questions are often concerned with achievements or changes over time, such as describing the average age of students upon graduation from PhD programs.

Normative questions describe a current standard and compare it with the ideal standard or norm (Mertens, 2010). Current standards are often found in documents such as organizational bylaws or standing committee operating procedures. Normative questions provide insight into whether a select intervention is achieving a desired specific aim. Normative questions may explore whether prospective students respond more positively to standard on-site information sessions or newly initiated webinar information sessions.

Output/impact questions are designed to determine the overall effects of the nursing program (Kellogg Foundation, 2010). Output/impact questions are concerned with whether the anticipated outcomes are the result of the program (Blanchard, et al. 2013). An example of a question that seeks to determine a program's outcome is as follows: Do employers indicate that alumni of the advanced practice nursing program, one year postgraduation, have comparable or more advanced client assessment skills than advanced practice nurses who did not attend the school's program?

CREATING AND SELECTING HIGH-QUALITY SURVEY QUESTIONS

Questions included on the survey need to be guided by the survey's purpose and any associated objectives. Keeping questions focused on the purpose and intent of the survey helps to ensure that quality data are generated to address both program needs and concerns of key stakeholders. Creating and selecting high-quality survey questions is a collaborative and iterative process among members of the evaluation team. Generating quality data is highly dependent on the quality of questions created and selected for the survey. Quality questions have several common characteristics that are highlighted in Table 4.1.

Question Placement

Opening questions provide a first impression of the survey and set the tone for the remainder of the survey. Opening questions, in particular, must be easy to answer, straightforward, and descriptive, such as the following:

Are you currently working in an advanced practice role?

___Yes, full time (more than 32 hours/week)

___Yes, part time (17–32 hours/week)

___Yes, part time (1–16 hours/week)

___No, but looking for employment as a nurse

___Not employed as a nurse or seeking employment as a nurse

In addition, it is wise to avoid or limit sensitive topics (e.g., "How many of your peers do you estimate use illicit drugs?"). Respondents are sensitive to certain topics and may feel uncomfortable or self-conscious providing answers to related questions. Certain questions may be sensitive to some respondents but germane to the survey's objectives. A principal example may be demographic questions such as income, race, or gender that not all respondents are comfortable answering. Potentially sensitive questions can be placed at the end of the survey with one response option being "Decline to answer." Questions about related topics need to be placed in close proximity to one another.

To summarize, characteristics of good questions link unmistakably to the evaluation's purpose and related aims. Respondents need to be able to answer program evaluation questions definitively and within a reasonable time frame. The questions can reflect concerns that are relevant to the program and address the needs and concerns of key stakeholders.

Format Response Options

Questionnaires, a widely used method for collecting program evaluation data, are formal written instruments consisting of items in which the wording of both the questions and frequently the response options are predetermined. Wide variation exists among questionnaires in their degree of structure ranging from closed-ended questions

TABLE 4.1

Characteristics of Survey Questions

Characteristic	In Need of Revision	Discussion	Example of Revision
Clarity	Since graduation, how many *formal* presentations have you delivered?	To minimize confusion or misunderstanding, the simplest language must be used or clarification needs to be provided. *Formal* may be a term for which respondents have differing interpretations. In addition, respondents cannot determine if it matters where the presentations were delivered (e.g., work, place of worship).	Since graduation, how many poster or podium presentations have you delivered at professional organization meetings, workshops, or conventions?
Specific	How would you rate your overall participation in professional organizations?	Without being overly wordy, questions need to enable the respondent to determine to what the question is specifically referring. The sample question does not specify date parameters (e.g., since starting nursing school).	Since January 2015, how would you rate your overall participation in professional nursing organizations?
Unbiased	Publications are an *expectation* of professional nurses. Since graduating, how many publications have you authored or co-authored?	Leading terms may bias respondents' answers to questions. The word *expectation* in the example may influence respondents to overestimate their publication history. Typically, biased questions lead respondents to provide the most socially desirable response.	Since graduating, how many publications have you authored or co-authored?

(continued)

TABLE 4.1

Characteristics of Survey Questions (Continued)

Characteristic	In Need of Revision	Discussion	Example of Revision
Ordered	**Question 1:** Do you approve or disapprove of the way administration is handling their job? **Question 2.** Overall, are you satisfied with the way things are going in the School of Nursing today?	The placement of questions can have a greater influence on the answer than the choice of words. Evaluators need to be attentive that earlier questions, such as in the example, have the potential to influence responses in subsequent questions.	Consider separating questions that may influence other questions by inserting a question that may be more innocuous in between, for example: How satisfied are you with the physical plant?
Focused	To what extent did your clinical instructor assign manageable patient care loads and answer your questions?	Questions that contain more than one item are referred to as "double-barreled." Double-barreled questions address numerous issues in the question's stem but allow for only one specific answer.	1. To what extent did your clinical instructor assign manageable patient care loads? 2. To what extent did your clinical instructor answer your questions?
Positive	Students did not participate in Legislative Day at the State Capitol. ___No ___Yes (Note: A negative response to this question suggests that students *did participate* while a positive response suggest students *did not participate*).	Answering negative or double-negative questions tends to confuse respondents. Confusion is easily reduced by removing the negative words. Negative words must be removed from both the stem and answers.	Did students attend Legislative Day at the State Capitol?

TABLE 4.1

Characteristics of Survey Questions (Continued)

Characteristic	In Need of Revision	Discussion	Example of Revision
Succinct	Do you believe that parking conditions at our clinical sites are challenging or difficult because of the lack of parking spaces and distance you have to walk to the clinical site, or do you believe that the parking situation at the clinical sites is fine?	Respondents, whether deans, students or employers, have precious little time to devote to surveys. Long questions with superfluous detail only add to respondent burden. Questions need to address the point as quickly as possible with economy of words.	What is your opinion of parking at our clinical sites?
Balanced	On average, over the past year, how often did you attend a professional in-service? a. Weekly b. Monthly	A balance between the question and response ratio is important. An adequate range of responses is needed for respondents to select answers genuinely reflecting their experiences, beliefs, or behaviors. Good program questions encourage answers that provide for both broader scope and meaning rather than simple yes/no responses.	On average, over the past 12 months, how often did you attend a professional in-service? a. Once per week b. Once each month c. Twice a year d. Once a year e. Never

to open-ended questions. Structured formats rely on closed-ended questions that provide response options for respondents to select the item most closely matching their answer (Boulmetis & Dutwin, 2011). Three types of closed-ended questions are often used in program evaluation surveys; these include dichotomous, multiple choice, and Likert scales (Table 4.2).

TABLE 4.2

Types of Closed-Ended Questions

Response Option	In Need of Revision	Discussion	Example of Revision
Dichotomous	Have you ever used the School of Nursing's Media Center? A. Yes B. No	Yes/No options are efficient to answer and are reasonable to use when simple comparisons are needed. However, very few responses in program evaluation are dichotomous. Most responses in program evaluation have a higher level of complexity and require variation in responses. Yes/No options provide limited depth of understanding.	How helpful have you found resources in the School of Nursing's Media Center to be in supporting your educational goals? A. Extremely helpful B. Helpful C. Somewhat helpful D. Not helpful E. Never used
Multiple Choice (needs to include the following three elements): 1. Mutually exclusive	1. How much time did you spend each day studying for your NCLEX? a. 1–2 hours b. 2–4 hours c. 4 hours or more	Multiple choice questions are efficient to answer and excellent to use when factual information is sought. Respondents select from a fixed set of options, and the question may be designed so that the respondent can select only one option or multiple options. 1. All of the possible options for selection should be different from each other, that is, options should be mutually exclusive. Parallel responses are not needed. Nondistinct options tend to confuse respondents. Answers must be mutually exclusive and collectively exhaustive. The items on the left overlap and therefore are not mutually exclusive. The answers are not collectively exhaustive because they do not take into account respondents who study less than one hour.	1. How much time did you spend each day studying for your NCLEX? a. Less than an hour b. 1–2 hours c. 3–4 hours d. 4 hours or more

TABLE 4.2

Types of Closed-Ended Questions (*Continued*)

Response Option	In Need of Revision	Discussion	Example of Revision
2. Capture all possible responses	2. Are you currently working in an advanced practice role? a. Yes, part-time b. Yes, full-time c. Not working	2. Using the smallest number of categories possible, strive to include all appropriate respondents. "Other" is a reasonable category to use in case an appropriate option was omitted.	2. Are you currently working in an advanced practice role? a. Yes, full-time (more than 32 hours/ week) b. Yes, part-time (17–31 hours/ week) c. Yes, part-time (1–16 hours/ week) d. No, but looking for employ-ment as an APRN e. Not employed as an APRN nor seeking employ-ment as an APRN
3. Logical sequencing	3. What is your highest earned degree in nursing? a. PhD b. MSN c. DNP d. BSN e. ADN f. LPN/LVN	3. To reduce confusion and limit the possibility that respondents will overlook an option, all items must have logical ordering.	3. What is your highest earned degree in nursing? a. LPN/LVN b. ADN c. BSN d. MSN e. DNP f. PhD

BOX 4.1

Likert Scale Options

1	2	3	4	5	6
Strongly Disagree	Disagree	Neither Agree nor Disagree	Agree	Strongly Agree	Don't Know

Likert Scales

Likert scales were originally designed to measure opinions (Polit & Beck, 2012) and thus work best when evaluators are trying to determine attitudes, beliefs, or preferences. Most respondents are familiar with the Likert format and are comfortable with its use. The typical Likert scale has 5 to 6 points for selection, with the sixth being reserved for "don't know." Smaller Likert scales may not capture the respondent's ideal choice, while larger scales can lose significance because the difference between two points is diminished. For example: On a scale from 0 to 100, 0 being "no involvement" and 100 being "highly involved," rate your level of agreement or disagreement with the following statement: "I am involved with the School of Nursing's Alumni Association." A 6-point Likert scale, as seen in Box 4.1, would provide more precise information regarding perceived level of alumni involvement.

A description needs to be provided for each point on the Likert scale. If points are without description, respondents have difficulty determining the numeric point's meaning. Explicitly stated descriptions minimize the possibility of respondent confusion. A neutral category on a Likert scale, such as "neither agree nor disagree," is helpful to respondents who may be familiar with the topic but have no fixed opinion either way. Without a neutral category, respondents are forced to create an opinion. The "don't know" option differs from the neutral option in that "don't know" indicates that a respondent is unfamiliar with the topic or does not feel inclined to answer. As with other scales, Likert-scale options should be presented logically. The ordering sequence of options needs to remain consistent for all Likert items on the survey. For example, the continuum from *strongly disagree* to *strongly agree* should be used consistently for each Likert-scale item on the questionnaire.

Filter or Contingency Questions

Frequently, respondents are asked an initial question to determine if they are qualified or experienced to answer successive questions. For example, alumni may be asked: Have you participated in any research activities over the past year? If the answer is "yes," respondents will be asked to check those research activities that they have engaged in over the past year. If respondents select "no," they will be directed to the next question (Box 4.2).

BOX 4.2

Example of Filter Options

Indicate Type of Research Activity

Data Collector

Research Assistant/Associate

Research Consultant

Research Coordinator

Project Director

Co-Investigator

Principal Investigator

Developed/Developing a Research Proposal

Member of a Research Committee

Postdoctoral Studies

Other

Filter or contingency questions can become complex and, therefore, need to be used prudently. To avoid unnecessary complexity, it is wise to use no more than three levels (2 jumps) for any filter question.

Open-Ended Questions

Unstructured, or open-ended, questions provide respondents with a predetermined question and allow for composition of a meaningful narrative response. Open-ended questions allow respondents to create a free-form answer using their own words (Fitzpatrick et al., 2011). The following is an example of an open-ended question: "What aspects of the nursing program enhanced your confidence to function as a beginning registered nurse?"

Responses to open-ended questions may provide rich and detailed information not easily discovered in predetermined answers to close-ended questions. Open-ended questions can be designed to encourage respondents to elaborate on a reply rather than provide a one-word answer. "Did you learn new information in the intensive block session?" is an example of a *closed-open-ended* question. One way to transform the question to prompt an open-ended response would be, "Describe what you learned from attending the intensive block session."

Because open-ended questions are exploratory, they often serve as groundwork for developing key closed-ended questions on upcoming surveys. Open-ended responses help in illuminating and providing a clearer understanding of patterns found in numeric data.

For example, students may rate technology used in a distance course as less than optimal. On inspection of the narrative, it may not be the technology that is distressing students but instead the academic implementation associated with technology. For instance, students may be concerned that discussion boards are used to post assignments rather than engaging students in meaningful and profitable discussion about the week's topic.

While responses to closed-ended questions can be immediately calculated and interpreted, open-ended questions require time and resources for detection of themes and analysis of findings. Conventionally, closed-ended questions are the default for program evaluation surveys and are used more frequently than open-ended questions. Program evaluation surveys often include a few open-ended questions if deeper understanding is needed about certain topics. Additionally, open-ended questions are used to allow respondents to address any key areas that they thought were missed on the survey.

Time-Related Questions

Often, program evaluation questions require respondents to consider events that occurred within a specific time frame, such as number of continuing education programs attended over the past year. Time-related questions, which require counting events or occurrences, are often prone to error because of fallible respondent recall. Respondents may not remember a specific event or may be unable to connect recollections that they have in a logical sequence. "How many professional presentations (podium or poster) did you present over the past year?" is an example of a time-related question that may present recall challenges. There are useful question design strategies to assist respondents with more accurate time recall. First, provide a specific time frame. "How many professional presentations (podium or poster) did you present over the past year?" is problematic because last year can be interpreted in a variety of ways. For some respondents, "last year" may mean since January. For other respondents, "last year" may mean the last 12 months since receiving the survey. For faculty members, "last year" may mean from the beginning of the academic year. Providing a specific time frame may aid with recall and will standardize the time frame for all respondents. Modifying the question to read, "In the past year, meaning since September 1, 2015, how many professional presentations (podium or poster) did you present?" may provide adequate time reference to improve respondent recall.

Second, use shorter time frames for less notable events but longer time frames for more distinguished events. For example, "How many professional meetings did you attend in the past month?" is more amenable to accurate recall than inquiring about professional meetings attended over the past year. However, "How many awards did you receive over the past 12 months?" may yield reliable answers because of the importance and probable infrequency of the event.

Third, avoid overuse of time frame recall questions. Asking respondents to recall and compile numerous events into meaningful patterns becomes easily tiring and tedious. Weary respondents may guess at answers or completely avoid the question.

Fourth, using an average rather than a precise count may satisfy the survey data requirements and prove to be less taxing for the respondent. To illustrate, "On average, how many professional meetings do you attend in a month?" may provide the needed information and be less tedious for a respondent to answer.

Establishing Priorities for Question Selection

Drucker (2015) observed that the most serious evaluation mistakes are not the result of wrong answers but instead are the result of asking the wrong questions. The ultimate success of program evaluation is, in large part, a result of good program evaluation questions. Once the evaluation team has drafted a set of reasonable evaluation questions, criteria must be established for selecting the most useful of those questions for a particular survey. Good evaluation questions focus on key aspects of both program planning and implementation. Therefore, prioritizing the selection of evaluation questions is critical in addressing key program objectives and implementation strategies. To assist with establishing priorities for selecting high-quality questions, it is necessary to consider several criteria. While not a universally accepted checklist for prioritizing and selecting the most useful evaluation questions, the following criteria will be helpful in identifying questions to provide the most beneficial information: (1) appropriate linkage, (2) stakeholder engagement, (3) relevance, (4) feasibility, and (5) impact.

Linkage between the purpose of the evaluation and the question is of primary importance. Several questions may provide answers that are "nice to know" but only questions with direct linkage to the evaluation purpose need to be given priority for selection. If employers are surveyed as a source to *evaluate program outcomes*, it may be necessary to inquire about the ability of alumni to deliver high-quality care in complex situations. It may be nice to know their salary range, but such information would not likely link to the purpose of the survey. In determining appropriateness of fit, it is important to decide if the program's values are evident in the question. For instance, if the program values educating state-of-the-practice advanced practice registered nurses (APRNs), then questions reflecting the Commission on Collegiate Nursing Education Essentials of Master's Education in Nursing (American Association of Colleges of Nursing, 2011) and National Organization of Nurse Practitioner Faculties core competencies are a priority, easily identifiable within the question bank.

When setting priorities for question selection, it is important to consider what stakeholder group will use the survey information and for what purpose. Stakeholders are generally the primary data collection source (Stufflebeam & Shinkfield, 2007). Students, faculty, alumni, and employers are examples of key stakeholders. Questions can address relevant stakeholders' needs and interests, including those of men and other minority groups in nursing. Stakeholder engagement is essential for the development of optimal evaluation questions. Each evaluation question needs to be ascertained to determine if stakeholders were engaged to some degree in developing or critiquing the evaluation questions. Stakeholder engagement helps to ensure that those who will be directly affected by the evaluation are engaged in developing the most appropriate questions affecting their stakeholder group. Stakeholder engagement also ensures that similar stakeholders have a clear understanding of the question and may even be inclined to use the evaluation results (Stufflebeam & Shinkfield, 2007).

Relevance is assessed to determine if the answered questions will be useful to the program and its stakeholders. For instance, inquiring about marketability of services may be pertinent to alumni who are one year postgraduation, but would have minimal relevance to students just finishing their first year of the nursing program. Assessing for relevance helps to determine if the question is the best source of information or if other

---

BOX 4.3

Matrix for Prioritizing and Selecting Survey Questions

Using the scale below, prioritize how well each criterion is represented in the question:
1 = Not represented at all
2 = Needs improvement
3 = Satisfactory representation
4 = Thoroughly represented

QUESTION #	Priority Score	Comments
1. Appropriate linkage		
2. Stakeholder engagement		
3. Relevance		
4. Feasibility		
5. Potential for impact		

Total Priority Score:

- Does the question meet inclusion criteria of ≥3 on each section? ___Yes ___No
- Based on the Priority Score (≥15), does the question merit survey inclusion? ___Yes ___No
- If the question does not meet the criteria but merits inclusion, state the rationale for inclusion:

---

sources of information—such as program administration data, observation, or in-depth case study—may be more useful yet less costly to use.

Feasibility is assessed to determine if a question can be answered by a stakeholder with a high degree of accuracy. For example, many alumni may be able to answer "How is your performance perceived by your employer?"; however, the accuracy of those responses may be doubtful. Feasibility is also concerned with determining if a question can be answered efficiently and with undue burden on a stakeholder.

Impact reflects how well each individual question fits in combination with other questions. Impact is assessing if questions, in their entirety, provide adequate information for developing a clear picture of the survey's purpose. Impact also assesses if the question, in combination with other questions, provides stakeholders enough information to take action on identified program issues or concerns (Box 4.3).

Indicators

An indicator is the gauge, or measurement, that answers the evaluation question. An indicator is an expression of what the evaluators want to know or observe. Thus, an

Example of Measurable Indicator

Evaluation Question	Measurable Indicators
Indicate your participation in professional organizations in the past year (e.g., American Nurses Association, Sigma Theta Tau, American Association of Critical Care Nurses).	• Attend meetings • Member of a committee • Chair of a committee • Elected or appointed as an officer • Review board for professional journal • Editor of a professional journal • Other

indicator is the observable evidence of program accomplishments, desired changes, or attained growth. Professionalism is a phenomenon that many programs want to measure as an alumni outcome. Yet, professionalism is a multidimensional, complex concept that can be observed in a variety of ways. To adequately document a program's impact on professionalism, the activities that *indicate* professionalism must be identified. These indicators are then used as markers of success for the desired outcome. An example depicting indicators for scholarship is demonstrated in Box 4.4.

SUMMARY

Questionnaires are a well-accepted method for collecting program evaluation data. Frequently, evaluators and faculty choose to develop their own questionnaires. Writing and selecting relevant evaluation questions are critical in the process of achieving meaningful survey results. Program evaluation surveys that are program focused, well defined, and precise lead to a higher probability of receiving accurate information that can result in optimal decisions regarding a nursing program.

References

American Association of Colleges of Nursing (2011). *The essentials of master's education in nursing.* Retrieved from http://www.aacn.nche.edu/education-resources/Masters Essentials11.pdf.

Blanchard, R. D., Torbeck, L., & Blondeau, W. (2013). AM last page: A snapshot of three common program evaluation approaches for medical education. *Academic Medicine, 88*(1), 146. doi: 10.1097/ACM.0b013e3182759419.

Boulmetis, J., & Dutwin, P. (2011). *Research methods for the social sciences: ABCs of*

evaluation: Timeless techniques for program and project managers (3rd ed.). San Francisco: Jossey-Bass.

BookBrowse. (2015). BookBrowse's favorite quotes. Voltaire. Retrieved from https://www.bookbrowse.com/quotes/detail/index.cfm/quote_number/406/judge-a-man-.

Cizek, G. J. (2010). An introduction to formative assessment: History characteristics and challenges. In H. L. Andrade & Cizek, G. J. (Ed.), *Handbook of formative assessment* (pp. 3–17). New York: Routledge.

Dillman, D. A., Smyth, J. D., & Christian, L. M. (2014). *Internet phone mail and mixed methods: Tailored design method* (4th ed.). Hoboken, NJ: John Wiley & Sons.

Drucker, P. F. (2015). Peter F. Drucker quotes. Retrieved August 29, 2015, from http://www.goodreads.com/author/quotes/12008. Peter_F_Drucker

Facione, N. C., & Facione, P. A. (2008). *Critical thinking and clinical reasoning in the health sciences: An international multidisciplinary teaching anthology.* Millbrae, CA: California Academic Press.

Fitzpatrick, J. L., Sanders, J. R., & Worthen, B. R. (2011). *Program evaluation: Alternative approaches and practical guidelines.* Boston: Pearson Education.

Mertens, D. M. (2010). *Research and evaluation in education and psychology: Integrating diversity with quantitative, qualitative, and mixed methods* (3rd ed.). Thousand Oaks, CA: Sage.

National Organization of Nurse Practitioner Faculties. (n.d.). *Competencies for Nurse Practitioners.* Retrieved from http://www.nonpf.org/?page=14.

Pew Research Center (2015) *Questionnaire Design.* Retrieved from http://www.pewresearch.org/methodology/u-s-survey-research/questionnaire-design/.

Polit, D. F., & Beck, C. T. (2012). *Nursing research: Generating and assessing evidence for nursing practice* (9th ed.). Philadelphia: Wolters Kluwer/Lippincott Williams & Williams.

Rossi, P. H., Lipsey, M. W., & Freeman, H. E. (2004). *Evaluation: A systematic approach* (4th Ed.). Thousand Oaks, CA: Sage.

Stufflebeam, D. L., & Shinkfield, A. J. (2007). *Evaluation theory models and applications.* San Francisco: Jossey-Bass.

Stump, G. S., Husman, J., & Brem, S. K. (2012). The nursing student self-efficacy scale: Development using item response theory. *Nursing Research, 61,* 149–158. doi: 10.1097/NNR.0b013e318253a750

W.K. Kellogg Foundation (2010). *W.K. Kellogg Foundation Evaluation Handbook.* Battle Creek, MI: W.K. Kellogg Foundation.

5

Developing a Systematic Program Evaluation Plan for a School of Nursing

Lynne Porter Lewallen, PhD, RN, CNE, ANEF

N urse educators evaluate every day. The first type of evaluation that educators think of is classroom and clinical evaluation of students. Nurse educators routinely do self-evaluations and peer evaluations, and administrators evaluate faculty and staff. But for some reason, when it comes to program evaluation, the whole process can seem foreign. Systematic program evaluation (SPE) is critical for program improvement as well as adherence to regulatory and accreditation standards. This chapter discusses the rationale for SPE and how to get started in creating a program evaluation plan or revising an existing plan. Areas to include in a plan are described, and samples of actual evaluation plans from two nursing programs are used to illustrate strategies to evaluate selected criteria.

MOTIVATION FOR DEVELOPING A PROGRAM EVALUATION PLAN

With the busy schedule of a nurse educator, it can be difficult to find the motivation to begin developing a SPE plan. All the theories about motivating adults to do something describe the importance of intrinsic motivators—motivators from inside. We might develop an evaluation plan if we are told that it is required (extrinsic motivation), but are more likely to do it well and to sustain our efforts when we also have some intrinsic motivation. When working day-to-day in a nursing program, it is sometimes difficult to see the "big picture" of the program because we are busy with our daily activities. Program evaluation helps faculty, administrators, and other stakeholders view the program as a whole; there will never be sufficient time to do this unless there is motivation to make it a priority.

Systematic program evaluation can provide a databased rationale for making changes or not changing what is currently being done. Changes based on data are often better accepted and can result in program improvement. Motivational theory posits that internal motivators are more important than external motivators in sustaining a behavior change for an individual (Deci & Ryan, 2000), and an internal motivator for every program is likely excellence. However, the fact remains that, in a busy educational environment, sometimes external motivators are more salient in the prioritization of workflow. As important as intrinsic motivators are, there also are many important extrinsic motivators for program evaluation, one of which is that meaningful program evaluation is required by regulators and accreditation bodies.

REGULATORY AND ACCREDITATION INFLUENCES IN PROGRAM EVALUATION

Nursing has many regulatory and accreditation influences, which are important to consider as the program develops a SPE plan. However, it is important to remember that the SPE belongs to the nursing program and needs to be useful in improving the program. If the plan is not useful, it will not be appropriate for accrediting and regulatory needs. If the faculty value the plan, they will be more likely to implement it and make changes based on the data collected. There are a number of regulatory and accreditation factors to consider when developing and using a SPE plan.

Regional Accrediting Bodies

With the exception of some stand-alone nursing programs, most nursing programs in the United States are located within parent institutions that are accredited by one of 7 regional accrediting bodies (U.S. Department of Education, 2015). Regional accrediting bodies are one of three categories of institutional accrediting agencies: regional, national faith-based, and national career-related, which are discussed in Chapter 7. Regional accrediting bodies—such as the Middle States Commission on Higher Education and the Southern Association of Colleges and Schools Commission on Colleges—accredit the parent institution, university, college, or community college in which the nursing program is located, enabling students to receive federal financial aid and transfer credits earned at the parent institution to other schools. These regional accreditors require that the parent institution collect and use evaluation data, such as student complaints, from each of its programs. The nursing program, and other units within the parent institution, need to collect data and report them to the parent institution as a whole.

Although regional accrediting bodies do not focus on individual programs and units within the institution, they require that the institution as a whole conduct program evaluation activities that examine the effectiveness and achievement of general college requirements and individual program outcomes. The nursing program is often required to participate in institution-wide quality enhancement plans (Southern Association of Colleges and Schools Commission on Colleges, 2015). These plans identify key issues from the institution's own assessment plan to improve student learning outcomes and should be reflected in the SPE in the school of nursing.

Nursing Accrediting Bodies

Nursing accreditation standards are important to consider when developing a program evaluation plan. The accrediting bodies for nursing education include the National

League for Nursing (NLN) Commission for Nursing Education Accreditation (CNEA) (NLN, 2015), currently seeking recognition from the U.S. Department of Education to accredit nursing programs; Accreditation Commission for Education in Nursing (ACEN, 2013); and Commission on Collegiate Nursing Education (CCNE, 2013). These are programmatic accreditors. All of these accrediting bodies have standards related to program outcomes. Specific required outcome measures vary, but all require evaluation of areas such as program outcomes, student learning outcomes, competencies of program graduates, and satisfaction of the employers of program graduates. The accrediting agencies require that certain data be collected, which would be reflected in the evaluation plan, and that the findings be used for program improvement. Accreditation is described further in Chapter 7.

State Boards of Nursing

Another agency affecting the evaluation of nursing programs is the state board of nursing. Approval of nursing programs by the state board is required in all states, although the criteria and processes vary. Some state boards of nursing require that nursing programs are accredited by national nursing accrediting bodies while others do not (Lewallen, DeBrew, & Stump, 2014), but all boards require evidence of program evaluation. Board of nursing requirements are often similar to those of nursing accrediting agencies but also may contain other specific requirements, all of which should be included in the SPE plan.

SUMMATIVE AND FORMATIVE EVALUATION

Program evaluation includes both summative, sometimes referred to as product, and formative, sometimes called process, components. Summative evaluation is an assessment of the completed program (Fitzpatrick, Sanders, & Worthen, 2011). For example, summative evaluation confirms whether the curriculum does what it says it will do in relation to the desired characteristics of the graduate. With summative evaluation, the program is evaluating its product. Questions asked in summative evaluation of a nursing program might include the following: Did we accomplish what we set out to accomplish? Were our students able to achieve the end-of-program outcomes? Was the program efficient in terms of time, personnel, and cost? Are our stakeholders (graduates, employers) satisfied with graduates' performance? Common areas measured with summative evaluation include end-of-program student satisfaction and licensing and certification examination results.

Formative evaluation of a nursing program occurs during the development of the program and its components (Fitzpatrick, Sanders, & Worthen, 2011). Formative evaluation is an opportunity to collect data to make changes before the program is completed. This type of evaluation can help determine if the best outcomes are being produced with the least expense in terms of time, effort, stress, finances, and use of resources. This is a detailed evaluation, which includes the evaluation of processes. With formative evaluation, changes can be made immediately. Questions asked in formative evaluation might include the following: Is this process working? Are our students progressing through the earlier courses in the curriculum? Formative evaluation allows for revision of courses and other changes in the program. Common areas measured with formative evaluation include results of achievement tests early in the nursing program and student satisfaction surveys.

DEVELOPING A SYSTEMATIC PROGRAM EVALUATION PLAN

When beginning to develop a SPE plan, it is important to decide what criteria for evaluation to include in it. An organizing framework can help with this decision. Some programs organize their SPE plans by accreditation or approval criteria. However, with this approach, the program also may want to evaluate additional areas. The sample evaluation plans included in Appendix A both base their SPE plans on accreditation standards.

Other nursing programs prefer to use an evaluation model to organize the SPE plan. Although evaluation models can be useful, there is always the risk that variables not in a particular model might be important for a program and may be missed if the model is used exclusively as the guide for evaluation (Stavropoulou & Stroubouki, 2014). There are many evaluation models in the literature, as discussed in Chapter 2. For example, a nursing program could use the CIPP (Context, Input, Process, Product) model (Stufflebeam, 2000) to guide development of its evaluation plan. The CIPP model examines intended ends and means as compared to actual ends and means. The four major areas of evaluation with this model are: (1) Context (intended ends), (2) Input (intended means), (3) Process (actual means), and (4) Product (actual ends). This model could be used to design an overall program evaluation and to assess a specific area of concern in the nursing program.

For context, what the program intends to accomplish, some areas of evaluation would include the mission, philosophy, setting, and requirements of internal and external stakeholders. Nurse educators would assess how well the nursing program philosophy and mission fit with those of the parent institution, how the curriculum meets professional standards, how the educational setting allows the nursing program to accomplish its goals, and if accreditation standards have been met. In the area of input, if the program design and resources accomplish program goals, areas of evaluation would include human and physical resources; student support systems; the design of the curriculum for all of the academic programs, including general education support and prerequisite courses; and the planned assessment methods for student achievement. For process, how the program design is actually working, evaluation areas would focus on whether the program is being implemented as planned, the curriculum is following the identified professional standards, resources are being used effectively, and teaching strategies are facilitating meeting the learning outcomes. In the area of product, how the actual program outcomes compare to the intended outcomes, some areas of evaluation would be if graduates are able to function in the roles for which they prepared and pass licensure and certification examinations, and if employers are satisfied with graduates' performance.

COMPONENTS OF A SYSTEMATIC PROGRAM EVALUATION PLAN

Once the evaluation criteria have been established, the plan should be structured to facilitate data gathering, analysis, and use. Both sample plans in Appendix A use a table format, which is a common method. The table can be customizable to the nursing program but, at minimum, should include the area of evaluation (commonly referred to as the criterion), expected level of achievement (ELA), person or group responsible for collecting the data, method of assessment, and time frame in which the data are collected

---

BOX 5.1

Areas to Include in Program Evaluation Document

The following areas should be included in your systematic program evaluation document:

Criterion (area of evaluation)
Expected level of achievement (ELA)
Person or group responsible for collecting the data
Method of assessment
Time frame
Actual data collected
Actions taken

(Box 5.1). Most SPE plans also include columns to record the actual data collected and actions taken as a result of analysis of those data. Generally, the plan document covers one academic year.

Areas of Evaluation

The areas of evaluation should include the accreditation requirements, but also may contain other areas of importance to the school of nursing. For example, a nursing program may evaluate if it is cost-effective to offer all or part of a course online. Frequently, nursing programs do not have processes in place to conduct cost-benefit analyses (Horne & Sandmann, 2012), but with the cost of nursing and higher education of concern, this is an area in which evaluation is important. Areas of evaluation to include in the plan are discussed further in the next section of this chapter.

Expected Level of Achievement

The ELA for each criterion should be developed thoughtfully. Sometimes, the ELA is prescribed by an external body. For example, the ACEN requires that the three-year average of the first-time pass rate on the National Council Licensure Examination (NCLEX) be at or above the national mean (ACEN, 2013), and the CCNE requires that the annual first-time NCLEX pass rate be at least 80% (CCNE, 2013). In this case, the program must meet a particular standard to remain in compliance with the accrediting agency. For other criteria, such as faculty scholarship, the program sets its own benchmarks. It is important to set benchmarks that are reasonable for the nursing program based on factors such as past performance. While it may be tempting to set high goals that the program is not likely to meet, the program will be continually in an area of deficit, explaining that benchmarks were not met.

A better plan is to establish a reasonable benchmark, with a long-term goal to increase it. Using faculty scholarship as an example, a long-term goal might be for each tenure-track faculty member to publish two articles in peer-reviewed journals per year. If the current baseline average is 0.5 articles per year, two for the next year is not a reasonable goal. Therefore, the first-year benchmark might be one per year, with the addition of an organized writing group for faculty to accomplish this goal. At the end of the year, evaluation data can lead the program to either increase the benchmark, if the goal was met, or improve the support systems for faculty if the goal was not met.

Responsible Person or Groups

The individuals or groups responsible for collecting the data should be identified for each criterion. It is important that this be specific: a general group such as "all faculty" may not result in data being collected in a systematic way. Some larger schools of nursing may have a specific person or office that collects all of the evaluation data; in smaller schools, the program director may have the primary responsibility. Ultimately, however, evaluation is more successful if the responsibility to collect data is shared among the faculty and administrators. Although one person or group may be responsible for the overall final audit of the SPE plan, including others in the data gathering and aggregation increases awareness of the importance of program evaluation and can lead to more useful measures being employed (Ellis & Halstead, 2012).

Another structure that can be employed for collecting evaluation data is the use of current committees in the school. For example, the curriculum committee might be responsible for collecting course evaluations, and a student affairs committee might be responsible for collecting student satisfaction data.

Method of Assessment

Another consideration is the method of assessment of each criterion. For example, if the program has a criterion about graduate satisfaction, then the instrument used to collect this information should have a question or a scale that specifically measures satisfaction. While this sounds self-evident, it is not uncommon for evaluation instruments to be designed in isolation from the criteria that they are intended to measure. An important point to remember is that there are many ways to evaluate whether the program is meeting the criteria in the SPE plan. It is not necessary to collect data using all possible evaluation methods; typically, one or two will suffice. Sometimes, accrediting agencies specify that both qualitative and quantitative measures be used, which should be reflected in the evaluation plan.

Time Frame

The evaluation plan should include a specified time frame in which the data are collected, such as at the end of each semester or academic year. By setting a specific time frame, it is easier to determine when to aggregate the data for reporting and action purposes.

Results

Many SPE plans also include a column for actual results. In that column, the data related to each criterion can be recorded for the academic year including the source of the data, such as the minutes of a particular meeting, which allows auditors to track the data and confirm the results. The program must have adequate documentation of both the data and decisions made. Minutes of meetings should have details about the discussions of aggregated outcomes and decisions based on those discussions. Decisions should be followed up with this process also documented. The discussions can be labeled in the meeting minutes with the evaluation plan criterion number, not only making it easy to track these discussions but also having the added benefit of keeping faculty aware of the SPE. For areas that are evaluated regularly, schools can set a certain time in the year for aggregating the data and reporting the results to stakeholders.

Actions Taken

The final column in the plan may contain the actions taken based on the evaluation. This column also can include plans for change, which should be specific to allow tracking the process of change during the next academic year. If the data show that the criterion is being met, this column may indicate that simply maintenance of the current process is needed.

STRUCTURE OF PROGRAM EVALUATION PLAN

Although the program evaluation plan should be tailored to your specific program, plans can look similar to one another. In Appendix A, two examples are provided of evaluation plans that illustrate the process and each of the components of evaluation. There is a sample from a community college that offers both a practical/vocational nursing education program and an associate degree nursing program, and another sample from a university-based school of nursing that has a Bachelor of Science in Nursing (BSN), RN-BSN, Master of Science in Nursing (MSN), Doctor of Nursing Practice (DNP), and Doctor of Philosophy (PhD) programs. It is often useful to have one document that contains the entire SPE plan. If the school of nursing offers multiple nursing programs, separate sections can focus on a particular program. However, having one document can ensure that nothing is missed.

Whether the program uses accreditation standards or an evaluation model to guide the structure of the evaluation plan, there are certain areas that all programs need to evaluate. These components include administration, faculty, students, curriculum, resources (including cost and efficiency), and program outcomes.

Administration

Nursing programs should be able to demonstrate how their program fits within the mission of the parent institution. This is often demonstrated with tables comparing the mission and vision of the parent institution with the mission, philosophy, and conceptual framework of the nursing program. Additional data to collect in the area of administration include budgetary support of the nursing program, both in comparison with other comparable programs in the institution and in relation to the work of the nursing program, for example, funding for adequate numbers of faculty. Documentation of faculty and student participation in the work of the institution and nursing program is necessary, and is often accomplished with a list of committee assignments.

When students are part of committees, it is important to document their attendance in the minutes and note instances in which student input was used, even if the students were not present at the meeting. One way that this can be accomplished is by discussing student feedback, formal or informal, about an issue and deciding on a course of action as a result of that feedback. Documentation of how students would be informed of the results of the discussion would "close the loop" (Banta & Blaich, 2011).

An additional area to consider is the integrity, or accuracy, of public information about the school of nursing. This involves clear communication about areas such as the admission and progression policies, grievance procedures, course offerings, and program plans. Public information can exist in many platforms, such as websites, catalogs, brochures, handbooks, and recruitment materials. One person could be assigned to monitor the consistency of information across these many venues. Integrity of public information should be assessed at least annually. Table A.1 in Appendix A provides an example of completed evaluation plans for faculty and student participation in program governance.

Faculty

Data collected related to faculty who teach in the nursing program include degrees held, progress toward advanced degrees, licensure, certifications, and continuing education. The goal is to document how faculty remain qualified for their positions. Qualifications of preceptors usually are described in this category as well. The amount of data about faculty can be difficult to aggregate in a way that is useful for the program. For this reason, it is helpful to identify a few key areas to evaluate and develop processes to make those data available for aggregation. Two areas that outside stakeholders often monitor closely are the degrees and licensure/certifications of faculty, as well as the amount and type of continuing education that faculty members complete. Generally, degrees, licensure and certification, and continuing education programs attended can be listed easily; more challenging can be the decision about whether the continuing education enabled faculty members to maintain their expertise.

Many nursing programs have position descriptions and guidelines for promotion and tenure that specify the expectations of faculty. If the data show that faculty members are not consistently meeting position expectations, areas to consider in the program evaluation might be if workloads are too high or if there are insufficient faculty development opportunities. This is a good illustration of how categories of evaluation are not mutually exclusive. An excessive workload may indicate a problem with administrative support in hiring additional nurse educators; a deficit in faculty development could indicate inadequate resources for professional development, a lack of time for faculty to attend continuing education, or a lack of offerings in the area. Table A.2 in Appendix A provides an example of how two programs assess faculty expertise.

Students

Areas to evaluate concerning students are the availability of student services, including services for students who learn online or at distant sites, maintenance of student records including financial aid records, and clear explanation of student policies. Formative evaluation is especially important in the area of students. There should be mechanisms in place for students to express concerns quickly to resolve small problems before they escalate. Programs also should evaluate how student complaints are handled to make sure that students receive due process. This is a requirement of regional and nursing accrediting bodies; parent institutions frequently monitor this process for each unit within the institution. Table A.3 in Appendix A is an example of how programs assess the student complaints process.

Curriculum

Important areas to include in a SPE related to the curriculum are an assessment of how the curriculum incorporates professional standards and practice realities, how each course is evaluated and the relationship of that process to the evaluation of the overall curriculum, and how clinical sites contribute to students' ability to meet course and program student learning outcomes. Data to monitor include the minutes of course and curriculum committee meetings, clinical site evaluation forms, students' performance on standardized tests as a reflection of how the curriculum meets national norms, employers' satisfaction with graduates as a reflection of how the curriculum addresses practice realities, and student and faculty evaluation of courses for both formative and summative purposes. It is critical to retain minutes of all meetings at which curriculum matters are discussed—these provide documentation for the evaluation plan and a record of decisions about the curriculum. Accrediting bodies require that faculty members be involved in the development, evaluation, and revision of the curriculum, an area in which documentation is frequently lacking. Table A.4 in Appendix A provides an example of how programs assess faculty participation in curriculum development, evaluation, and revision.

Resources

The category of resources is broad and includes all of the human, physical, learning, and fiscal resources that affect the nursing program. This is an area that is often neglected in SPEs because resources may not have a natural end point such as the end of a program or an academic year. Human resources to be assessed include adequacy of both faculty and staff such as academic advisers, information technology (IT) support, and clerical personnel. Examples of records to maintain include number of student visits to advisers, number of consultations for IT support and typical wait time for both faculty and students, and typical lead time required for faculty members to receive clerical support. Physical resource assessment includes areas such as classroom size and technology adequacy, faculty office adequacy, clinical site effectiveness in providing opportunities to practice necessary skills, and clinical laboratory and simulation opportunities (Appendix A, Table A.5). Learning resources can include the library, including online resources, and the availability of tutoring. Fiscal resources include funding for faculty positions, salary increases, staff support, faculty development and travel, and equipment purchases. If the school of nursing offers programs at a distance, it is important to assess resources that contribute to both student and faculty success in this learning format.

Program Outcomes

Program outcomes are commonly measured as part of a SPE. Outcomes measurement relies heavily on external sources of information such as surveys of employers, thus access to those sources is an important consideration. To effectively evaluate achievement of program outcomes, they need to be well defined, and multiple measures should be used. Internal measures might include an assessment of a comprehensive project, such as a portfolio, capstone project, thesis, or dissertation. Examples of external measures are first-time pass rates on licensure and certification examinations, scores on comprehensive tests, and employer satisfaction with the graduates' performance.

One type of data that is collected in this area is the length of time for students to complete the program. Accrediting agencies, boards of nursing, and parent institutions monitor program completion rates and may have specific benchmarks to which programs are held. Often, nursing programs document the percentage of students who complete the program within the published length of time and then how many finish at 150% of that length of time.

Data collected from graduates of the program include their perceptions of their achievement of program outcomes; satisfaction with the program including courses, quality and responsiveness of the faculty, clinical experiences, learning resources, and the grievance and complaint process; and readiness to assume the role for which they were prepared. Typically, this information is collected near the end of the program. If students have been offered a position, it is valuable to collect employment information.

Data collected from alumni include their achievement of program outcomes; their satisfaction with the program; information about the type of position that they obtained and preparation for it; licensure and certifications; progression to advanced degrees; and leadership roles, publications, and professional presentations, among others. Alumni information is collected typically at a time point between 6 months and one year after graduation, although some schools of nursing also collect data at later intervals.

The employers of graduates of the program can provide important information about the graduates' ability to function in the position for which they were hired and the satisfaction of employers with the graduates' readiness for entry into practice. Other general information that can be gathered from employers includes new skills being required of graduates and areas in which they need extensive orientation; this type of information may be useful to the program in making decisions about curriculum revisions.

Table A.6 in Appendix A provides an example of outcomes data specified on an evaluation plan. In this example, aggregated data are reported, which allow faculty to assess the program's achievement of the overall criterion. This example also illustrates the necessity of analyzing not only the data, but the process of evaluation itself, sometimes referred to as meta-evaluation (Stavropoulou & Stroubouki, 2014). While the results in this example are positive, in some programs the response rate for the surveys is low, leading to concern about the accuracy of the data given the small sample size. The risk of a biased sample is high, and the program may not have enough data on which to base conclusions and revisions.

CHALLENGING AREAS TO EVALUATE: GATHERING OUTCOMES DATA FROM GRADUATES, ALUMNI, AND EMPLOYERS

Surveys are a common method of collecting data from graduates, alumni, and employers. They allow the program to collect specific data from a large number of respondents and do so quickly. However, low response rates for surveys are a common problem (Story et al., 2010). Electronic surveys may yield a better response rate than mailed surveys because they are faster to complete; however, email addresses change frequently and bounce-backs may be common. It is important to obtain students' personal email addresses before they graduate from the program, even if the institution allows them to keep their student email addresses.

Another way to collect data from graduates is through focus groups. Although focus groups include fewer people than with a survey, you may obtain richer data for use in program evaluation. For example, focus groups of new graduates were of value in identifying areas of the curriculum that were most and least helpful in achieving the program outcomes (Nugent & LaRocco, 2014). Focus groups could be held between the last day of class and graduation, when memories are "fresh" but grading is completed, or at times when orientation groups meet at the largest employers of graduates of the program. Social media also can be used to collect data about program outcomes and provide access to surveys. Facebook groups have been used to seek comments about the nursing program and include links to online surveys (Lewallen, 2015). One school of nursing reported an increase in alumni survey response from 0 to 52% by using Facebook (Story et al., 2010). Nursing programs may be hesitant to use social media in pedagogy (Schmitt, Sims-Giddens, & Booth, 2012) as well advertising and evaluating their programs; however, this can result in missed opportunities for communication with alumni.

Many graduates keep in touch with one or two faculty members and may provide information about new positions, graduate school, and experiences that would be helpful for the program in considering improvements. If there were an established mechanism for faculty to easily document that information, it could be aggregated for program evaluation purposes.

In addition to contacting alumni by mail, email, or social media, they can be reached in other ways, especially if they tend to be concentrated in one geographic area. The nursing program can set up tables at major employers at lunchtime to talk to alumni; this strategy can be used to gather employment data, collect brief survey data, and recruit alumni for higher degree programs if offered by the school. This same strategy could be employed at nursing organization or community meetings; an alumni reception or table can facilitate gathering of data. Events held by the parent institution also provide a place to make contact with alumni for program evaluation. If the parent institution has an alumni association, that group may be a source of alumni contact and employer information.

To collect data from employers, similar strategies can be used as described earlier for alumni. Frequently, employers will attend similar nursing conferences and community events as alumni and can be reached in the same way. Other strategies to reach employers are periodic focus groups for lunch and contact at regular meetings that agency representatives attend, such as clinical coordination meetings (Lewallen, 2015). Most nursing programs have advisory boards, of which alumni and employers of graduates may be members; that group can provide valuable information and may have other contacts to facilitate gathering a wider sampling of data. It is also recommended to reach out to alumni who employ graduates of the program. Although it is not possible to contact every employer of every graduate, important data can be collected by speaking to smaller groups that are representative of the types of agencies that employ program graduates.

EVALUATE PROCESS

Finally, it is important to evaluate periodically the SPE plan. As faculty, administrators, and other stakeholders use the plan, they should identify areas in which the criteria need to be changed and measures that are not providing the needed data. As accreditation standards change, the plan may need revision. The program evaluation plan should be a "living document"—one that is used and amended as necessary to serve your program's purposes.

SUMMARY

Program evaluation is critical to ensuring the success of the nursing program, but it must be systematic and planned. If program evaluation can be integrated into the normal workflow of the program, it is less burdensome and will generate data for program improvement. When beginning to develop a SPE plan, it is important to decide what criteria for evaluation to include in it. An organizing framework can help with this decision. Some programs organize their SPE plans by accreditation or approval criteria; however, with this approach the program also may want to evaluate additional areas. Whether the program uses accreditation standards or an evaluation model to guide the structure of the evaluation plan, there are certain areas that all programs need to evaluate. These areas include administration, faculty, students, curriculum, resources, and program outcomes.

References

Accreditation Commission for Education in Nursing. (2013). *Accreditation Manual. Standards and Criteria.* Atlanta: Author. Retrieved from http://www.acenursing.org/accreditation-manual/

Banta, T. W., & Blaich, C. (2011) Closing the assessment loop. *Change: The Magazine of Higher Learning, 43*(1), 22–27. doi: http://dx.doi.org/10.1080/00091383.2011.538642

Commission on Collegiate Education in Nursing. (2013). *Standards for Accreditation of Baccalaureate and Graduate Degree Nursing Programs.* Washington, DC:

Author. Retrieved from http://www.aacn.nche.edu/ccne-accreditation/Standards-Amended-2013.pdf

Deci, E. L., & Ryan, R. M. (2000). The "what" and "why" of goal pursuits: Human needs and the self determination of behavior. *Psychological Inquiry, 11,* 227–268.

Ellis, P., & Halstead, J. (2012). Understanding the Commission on Collegiate Nursing Education accreditation process and the role of the continuous improvement progress report. *Journal of Professional Nursing, 28,* 18–26. doi:10.1016/j.profnurs.2011.10.004

Fitzpatrick, J. L., Sanders, J. R., & Worthen, B. R. (2011). *Program evaluation: Alternative approaches and practical guidelines* (4th ed.). Boston: Pearson.

Horne, E. M., & Sandmann, L. (2012). Current trends in systematic program evaluation of online graduate nursing education: An integrative literature review. *Journal of Nursing Education, 51*, 570–578. doi: 10.3928/01484834-20120820-06

Lewallen, L. P. (2015). Practical strategies for nursing education program evaluation. *Journal of Professional Nursing, 31*, 133–140. http://dx.doi.org/10.1016/j.profnurs.2014.09.002

Lewallen, L. P., DeBrew, J. K., & Stump, M. R. (2014). Regulation and accreditation requirements for preceptor use in undergraduate education. *Journal of Continuing Education in Nursing, 45*, 386–390. doi: 10.3928/00220124-20140826-01

National League for Nursing. (2015). *National League for Nursing CNEA Mission and Values.* Retrieved from http://www.nln.org/accreditation-services/the-nln-commission-for-nursing-education-accreditation-%28cnea%29

Nugent, E., & LaRocco, S. (2014). Comprehensive review of an accelerated nursing program: A quality improvement project. *Dimensions of Critical Care Nursing, 33*, 226–233. doi: 10.1097/DCC.0000000000000054

Southern Association of Colleges and Schools Commission on Colleges. (2015). *General Information on the Reaffirmation Process.* Retrieved from http://www.sacscoc.org/genaccproc.asp

Schmitt, T. L., Sims-Giddens, S. S., & Booth, R. G. (2012). Social media use in nursing education. *Online Journal of Issues in Nursing, 17*(3).

Stavropoulou, A., & Stroubouki, T. (2014). Evaluation of educational programmes—the contribution of history to modern evaluation thinking. *Health Science Journal, 8*, 193–204.

Story, L., Butts, J. B., Bishop, S. B., Green, L., Johnson, K., & Mattison, H. (2010). Innovative strategies for nursing education program evaluation. *Journal of Nursing Education, 49*, 351–354. doi:10.3928/01484834-20100217-07

Stufflebeam, D. L. (2000). The CIPP model for program evaluation. In G. F. Madaus, M. Scriven, & D. L. Stufflebeam (Eds.). *Evaluation models: Viewpoints on educational and human services evaluation.* Norwell, MA: Kluwer Academic Publishers.

U.S. Department of Education. (2015). *The Database of Accredited Post-Secondary Institutions and Programs.* Retrieved from http://ope.ed.gov/accreditation/Agencies.aspx

6

Ensuring Quality of Evaluation Data

Teresa Shellenbarger, PhD, RN, CNE, ANEF

Nurse educators need to carefully consider a variety of factors when conducting assessment and evaluation of nursing programs. Faculty face many choices about data collection and rely on systematically collected quality data to make good decisions. This chapter provides an overview of data and data sources frequently used in program evaluation. Psychometric considerations of reliability and validity are addressed, as well as other internal and external factors that impact data quality. The chapter continues with a discussion of types and forms of data collection approaches used in nursing program assessment and evaluation. Both quantitative and qualitative data collection approaches are discussed. The chapter also describes existing assessment tools that are available for program evaluation. Since it is imperative for faculty to capture data from key stakeholders, suggestions for methods of gathering these data are included in the chapter along with innovative approaches for technology use to assist this process.

DATA AND DATA SOURCES

When planning for data collection, faculty make many decisions. They need to consider the questions that need to be answered or the purpose of the assessment and gather data that will provide meaningful information. The type of program (e.g., prelicensure, second degree, advanced practice nursing) and the reason for collecting program assessment data (for program improvement or to provide data for local, regional, national, or specialty accreditation) become important considerations. Often, data collection decisions are influenced by regulations and guidelines from external bodies such as specialized nursing accreditation agencies or state boards of nursing. These decisions also may be influenced by national, regional, or state organizations that provide overall institutional review and accreditation. The parent institution may require specific information from the nursing program, thus impacting decisions about data collection. In addition, the unique needs of the program and students influence decisions about data collection and

---

BOX 6.1

Sources of Data Used for Nursing Program Assessment and Evaluation

Course Evaluations
Examinations (faculty-made or standardized)
Focus groups
Institutional records and reports
Interviews
Nationally gathered records and reports such as National Council of State Boards
of Nursing and National Survey of Student Engagement reports
Portfolios
Projects, papers, assignments
Standardized examinations
Structured observation
Surveys

---

selection of data sources. Faculty knowledge, expertise, skills, beliefs, and values impact data collection choices as well. Last, fiscal, personal, and material resources and available support play an important role in decision-making about data collection. Faculty may have many ideas about possible data collection approaches, but if resources are not available to support the proposed data collection strategy, alternative approaches may need to be considered. All of these factors influence the decision-making about data collection for nursing program assessment and evaluation, and may ultimately influence the quality of the evidence.

Because program decisions are based on the data collected, faculty need to ensure that the data provide an accurate and unbiased representation of the students and the program. A variety of data sources are typically used by nursing programs as part of their program evaluation plan (Lewallen, 2015). Many schools select an array of qualitative and quantitative data-collection approaches and triangulate the elements to ensure that they capture the needed information (Eder, 2014). Box 6.1 provides a listing of some common data sources used by nursing programs for assessment and evaluation. More information about data and data sources is provided later in this chapter.

Because of the importance of the data for program decision-making, nursing programs should gather input from various perspectives while also addressing key evaluation questions. Programs gather data from a variety of stakeholders including students, faculty, clinical partners, employers, and alumni to ensure a comprehensive and representative review of the program (Horne & Sandman, 2012). Box 6.2 offers a listing of potential providers of nursing program assessment and evaluation data.

PSYCHOMETRIC CONSIDERATIONS

Another important factor when making decisions about data collection for nursing program evaluation purposes involves psychometric considerations. Some important psychometric principles are discussed so that readers understand the impact of these

---

BOX 6.2

Providers of Nursing Program Assessment and Evaluation Data

Administrators
Advisory groups
Agencies (state boards of nursing, nursing accreditation bodies)
Alumni
Clinical agency (staff, preceptors, supervisors, and employers)
Faculty
Institution (in which nursing program is housed)
Students

---

issues. Gathering psychometrically sound data that are valid and reliable will help to enhance confidence in the findings.

Reliability

One important psychometric consideration involves ensuring reliability. Although some people may believe that reliability refers to the consistency of the data, this is an inaccurate interpretation of reliability. Instead, reliability refers to how closely measured scores are consistent with differences in their true scores (Furr & Bacharach, 2014). In other words, if the measurement is completed at different times, would similar results emerge? Is the measurement repeatable?

Four types of reliability are commonly reported: stability, equivalence, internal consistency, and interrater reliability. Stability usually involves a test-retest with correlations of those scores (Oermann & Gaberson, 2014). High reliability scores or correlations (close to 1.0) are preferred. Another type of reliability is equivalence, but this measure may not be used in program evaluation unless an alternate or parallel form of an assessment is available. The most commonly used statistic to measure internal consistency, the third type of reliability, usually involves a Cronbach's coefficient alpha (Pallant, 2013). Coefficient scores can range from 0.0 to 1.00, but, generally, nurse educators would be satisfied with a Cronbach's alpha value of 0.70 or 0.80 given the limited risks associated with decision-making based on the results (Furr & Bacharach, 2014; McDonald, 2014). The last type of reliability that may be important to consider, particularly for open-ended assessments, is interrater reliability. If two or more raters are evaluating an item, consistency is established when there is agreement in their rating.

Educators need to be aware that a number of factors can influence the internal consistency results such as the length of the tool, similarity of the assessment items, variability of the students, and sample size. Additionally, if items are poorly constructed or hard to understand, there can be an impact on reliability. Faculty conducting a nursing program evaluation should take steps to ensure reliability and foster quality data collection.

Validity

Another important psychometric consideration involves validity. This refers to truthfulness or determination of whether the tool or test measures what it is supposed to. Like reliability, it is not the tool or test that is assessed as valid but the accurate interpretations of the assessment. In the past, evaluators used terms such as face, content, criterion, or construct validity, but the more popular and contemporary approach is to discuss construct validity (Furr & Bacharach, 2014). This type of validity indicates whether the scores are reflective of the construct being measured. In other words, can the tool or test distinguish between those with certain characteristics from those without it (Fink, 2015)? For example, when interpreting results from a tool that measures clinical reasoning, the results would accurately identify those with clinical reasoning skills and not some related concept.

Similar to reliability, a number of factors can impact validity and include the content assessed and structure of the assessment. For some topics, particularly sensitive issues, participants may want to provide a socially desirable response, which may not be valid. Nurse educators can try to limit this type of response and minimize the threat to validity by ensuring confidentiality and anonymity of responses (Sue & Ritter, 2012). Sample size and sample selection may also affect validity; therefore, faculty conducting program evaluations should use large representative samples when possible to lessen the impact or threat to validity (Polit & Beck, 2012). Ensuring that questions are complete and provide sufficient and appropriate response options also will help to ensure validity.

OTHER FACTORS THAT IMPACT DATA QUALITY

There are a variety of other factors that impact data collection and may ultimately influence the quality and quantity of data collected. Some of these factors are internal issues directly related to the program and faculty. Others are factors that are external to the program related to data collected from outside of the institution.

Internal Factors

A variety of internal factors—such as the students, faculty, and program resources—may have an impact on the data collection and ultimately the quality of the data. Demographics of the students in the program may influence decisions made about data collection strategies. Student enrollment status (part-time vs. full-time), external demands on student time (work, family), type of program (prelicensure, second degree, advanced practice, doctoral), skill set (technology access and use), motivation, as well as other factors may influence the data collection approach selected. These factors also may influence student willingness to participate in nursing program evaluation activities such as surveys, focus groups, and interviews. Are students motivated to assist faculty and invest the time to participate in the activities, particularly if they occur outside of class meeting times?

Another factor that may impact willingness to participate involves the protection of participants' identity and responses. Faculty should assess if students are comfortable providing information to them or if neutral parties should be used for data collection activities. Faculty need to protect the rights of students during data collection and analysis. Strategies to safeguard students include removing identifying information from data, protecting sensitive information, and assuring confidentiality. Steps should be taken to ensure that participants provide honest, accurate, and appropriate information. Data collection tools should be created to limit response bias, decrease social desirability of responses, and prevent random or careless responses. Providing an appropriate environment free of distractions is also helpful in lessening the impact of internal factors. Last, faculty should be sensitive to survey length and timing of administration as participants may get tired and not pay attention during lengthy surveys. This inattention leads to survey fatigue, which may influence respondent results and lead to poor data quality (Ben-Nun, 2008). Later in this chapter, additional ethical concerns related to program evaluation are discussed.

Faculty skills and expertise also influence data collection and the resultant quality of the data. An important consideration is whether faculty have the knowledge and skills to complete both qualitative and quantitative data collection and analysis. Do they have the technological skills to construct electronic surveys, create databases, and analyze data with spreadsheets or statistical programs? If not, are there campus resources or support services that can assist them? Can workshops and training be provided to help faculty develop the skill set needed for data collection and analysis, and for program evaluation? In some schools, administrators or designated faculty oversee nursing program evaluation activities as part of their workload. In other schools, all faculty participate in these assessment and evaluation activities. Regardless of the approach used, those planning, implementing, and evaluating program data need to have the necessary skill set to carry out these activities.

Another internal factor that may impact the data quality involves resources. Does the institution have the financial resources to purchase standardized surveys, or is data collection reliant on faculty-developed materials? Is there staff support available to assist with clerical activities such as transcription of interviews and data entry? Are resources available to conduct the best type of data collection and analysis? Internal factors, such as those discussed earlier, become important considerations for nursing program evaluation.

External Factors

A variety of factors external to the institution can impact data collection and analysis. Participants external to the institution—such as employers, preceptors, and advisory group members—may influence the quality of the data that are collected. Using simple and straightforward data-collection approaches will assist in obtaining needed information. External stakeholders will appreciate brevity, organization, clear directions, easy completion, and well-constructed assessment materials (Sauter, Gillespie, & Knepp, 2012). Reaching the appropriate stakeholder for data collection is another important factor to consider. Some schools send graduates an alumni survey and ask that the former student forward the survey to the employer for completion. This approach frequently results in a low response rate, as it requires reliance on the graduate to forward materials and requires the employer to take the time to complete and return the survey (Sauter et al., 2012). Taking steps to distribute materials to the right person and making return of the materials easy will be appreciated by participants and may improve response rates. Simple steps such as including a self-addressed, prestamped envelope can facilitate responses (Dillman, Smythe, & Christian, 2014).

Timing of the data collection is another important external factor to consider. Faculty should ensure that those asked to complete evaluation materials have adequate time for the assessment and experience to evaluate the topic of inquiry. Also, faculty should avoid data collection near holidays and other busy times. Administrators and faculty responsible for program evaluation should consider these internal and external factors to help ensure the quality and quantity of data obtained.

TYPES OF DATA COLLECTION APPROACHES

Most programs use a variety of data collection approaches to gather comprehensive information for evaluation purposes. When making decisions about data collection, faculty should consider what data are already accessible and available in the nursing program. Using available institutional information may save cost and time, but faculty should review the data to ensure that they meet program evaluation needs. If existing instruments are not available, faculty may need to consider adapting an instrument or developing a new one. Polit and Beck (2012) caution that creating new valid and reliable instruments can be challenging, particularly for those without experience in tool development. However, many programs still choose to use locally developed surveys and tests more than standardized evaluations (Banta & Palomba, 2015). If a new tool needs to be developed, or an existing tool is modified, faculty should take steps to ensure that it is appropriate for answering the evaluation questions. These steps are provided in Box 6.3.

Nurse educators, similar to nurse researchers in practice, rely heavily on structured self-reporting either through interviews or questionnaires (Polit & Beck, 2012, p. 297). These self-reported measures may help to assess opinions, attitudes, actions, feelings, or beliefs. When designing self-reported measures, faculty should consider the use of either open- or closed-ended questions.

BOX 6.3

Steps in Tool Development

1. Set boundaries for the evaluation, including the type of measure and information to be collected.
2. Define the assessment topic.
3. Outline the content.
4. Select response choices.
5. Choose rating scale.
6. Review the measure with experts and potential users by pretesting.
7. Revise as needed.
8. Finalize the format (layout, directions).
9. Pilot test.
10. Revise as needed.

Adapted from Fink, A. (2015). *Evaluation fundamentals: Insights into program effectiveness, quality, and value*. Thousand Oaks, CA: Sage.

Open-Ended Questions

One type of self-report involves open-ended questions. These free-response questions do not give respondents answers from which to choose, but rather are phrased for respondents to explain their answers and reactions in their own words. Typically open-ended questions begin with words such as "Why" and "How" or phrases such as "Tell me about...." Often, they are not technically a question but rather a statement that asks for a response. Open-ended questions are used frequently when data cannot be placed easily into categories. For example, free-response questions are used to assess complex and unclear issues, or when answers cannot be anticipated. Open-ended questions are frequently incorporated into interviews, focus groups, or as a free-text response on questionnaires. This format provides for rich descriptive data but makes it challenging and time-consuming for faculty to analyze and interpret responses due to the varied nature of the responses. Regardless of the potential obstacles, open-ended questions offer one option for data collection and yield useful nursing program evaluation data.

Closed-Ended Questions

Another type of self-reported measure, the closed-ended question, encourages a short or single-word answer or forced-response option. Due to their structured nature and set of finite answers, closed-ended questions limit respondents' answers, as they are forced to choose from either a set of dichotomous answers such as yes/no, true/false, forced-choice items, multiple choice, or a ranking of item options, as in Likert-scale responses. Closed-ended questions might be used in program evaluation when possible answers are known, when information can be quantified, or because of their efficient method of data collection and analysis. They are often easier to analyze, may be more specific, and take less time for users to complete than open-ended questions. However, closed-ended questions may be more difficult to construct because the developer needs to know all the possible answers or response choices. Additionally, some critics have argued that using closed-ended questions may not represent the true feeling of respondents and have the possibility of omitting possible response categories. Box 6.4 offers some examples of open- and closed-ended question stems that can be helpful in guiding question creation.

BOX 6.4

Examples of Program Assessment Questions

Examples of open-ended questions
    Tell me about _____.
    How did you _____?
    How does ____affect ____?

Examples of closed-ended questions
    How often have you _____?
    Rank the most frequently used _____.
    How many hours of _____ have you completed?
    Are you satisfied with _____?

FORMS OF DATA COLLECTION

Regardless of the type of question, data can be obtained in a variety of formats. Some commonly used approaches include in-person, mailed, mobile, and telephone surveys; face-to-face interviews; and focus groups. Each strategy brings unique advantages and disadvantages. Table 6.1 provides an overview of each of these forms of data collection as well as some special considerations for faculty when they choose their method of data collection.

TABLE 6.1

Comparison of Data Collection Methods

Method	Advantages	Disadvantages	Considerations
In-person survey	Can distribute to and collect quickly and efficiently from groups. Researcher can be available to answer questions. Personal contact can positively influence response rate.	Gaining access to groups can be challenging.	Implement strategies to minimize data collector influence on responses.
Mail surveys	Can reach a large audience and geographic dispersion. Respondents can answer when convenient. No bias because there is no personal contact. Single researcher can complete the project.	Sometimes surveys are not completed or returned. Responses may be biased due to self-selection of completion. No one is available to explain or answer questions. Typically low response rates, especially if there are no incentives or methods to promote participation; use of advance letters, follow-up contacts, incentives, and a variety of other procedures can increase response rates. Need to wait for responses to be returned. No control over environment when completing. Costs for duplication/distribution (mailing).	Better to use for respondents with interest in the subject. Use techniques that enhance physical appearance of survey and promote responses (e.g., stamped, addressed return envelope) (Dillman, Smythe, & Christian, 2014). Use follow-up reminders to enhance response rates.

TABLE 6.1

Comparison of Data Collection Methods (*Continued*)

Method	Advantages	Disadvantages	Considerations
Online/ mobile/ web-based surveys	Rapid return of responses. Real time access. Can reach a large number of people. Can easily track results and respondents. Is economical. Is convenient for users.	Only reaches users with access to technology. May have low response rates (Polit & Beck, 2012).	Survey should be viewable from all electronic devices (mobile phones, iPad, laptops, and so on).
Telephone surveys	Easy to adapt to needs of respondents. Interviewer can explain questions if needed. Interviewer can probe for additional information and explanations.	Cost Human resources needed to conduct telephone surveys. May have difficulty reaching participants due to call screening. People have limited time when available. Phone contacts may not have been updated.	Current phone numbers are needed, which may not always be accessible.
Face-to-face interview	Can establish rapport with respondent. Can explore topics more fully with probing and questioning techniques. Allows for use of respondents' own words and not predetermined categories. High response rates (Polit & Beck, 2012)	Time needed to arrange and complete interview. Interviewer can impact responses. Transcription of audio files and data analysis can be time consuming.	Need interview guide and interviewer training.
Focus groups	Opinions and viewpoints can be obtained from multiple people at the same time. Allows for interaction among participants. Moderator can explore and clarify participant responses.	Participants may be uncomfortable expressing views in a group. Group members may be influenced by others in the group and strive to conform.	Consider selection of homogeneous groups. Carefully select moderator and data collection location to ensure neutrality. Use strategies to ensure participation of all members.

Quantitative Data Collection Approaches

Faculty need to make a decision about the type of data collection approach that they will use for program evaluation. Those making data collection decisions should consider the format that will provide the most useful data and gather data from a sufficient number of stakeholders. Given the advantages of closed-ended questioning approaches, quantitative surveys and questionnaires are frequently selected.

Either paper-and-pencil surveys administered in person or online electronic surveys are commonly used to gather program evaluation information. Faculty need to consider the survey instrument, sampling approach, and sample size when planning to use surveys. If there are no adequate existing surveys or if they do not meet program needs, then faculty will need to create a new survey. They should consider the recommendations found in Box 6.5 for tool development.

Another survey consideration involves the method of administration. Regardless if the survey is to be administered in-person, online, or by phone, some general principles apply. Faculty should consider the target audience and how to access them. If gathering survey responses from students, then either in-person distribution or online survey data collection methods may work best. Accessing data from sources away from the program's physical location may be best achieved by online or phone survey methods.

Sampling is another important consideration when using survey methods. Faculty should determine the approach used to select participants. Will convenience or probability sampling methods be used? Sample size also needs to be considered. Are all parties invited to participate? Regardless of the survey method used, faculty should consider alternatives and have a strong rationale for the choices made.

BOX 6.5

Considerations for Developing Program Evaluation Tools

Focus on a single item.
Do not ask questions that contain multiple components.
Include appropriate details.
Assess the relevant time period for accurate recall.
Ensure that statements are inclusive and without bias.
Avoid negatively worded statements.
Use simple, clear language and familiar words understood by the respondents.
Spell out acronyms.
Avoid jargon.
Ensure that grammar, spelling, and content are accurate.
Use selective combinations of boldface type, underlining, and capitals for emphasis.
Phrase questions in a nonthreatening, straightforward, and direct manner.
Ensure that the content and questions apply to the respondents.
Make choices mutually exclusive and not overlapping.
Have items reviewed by others prior to use.
Pretest and pilot test newly developed items.

Qualitative Data Collection Approaches

There are a variety of data collection approaches that use open-ended questioning and employ traditional qualitative research methods. The following section discusses some key considerations for program evaluators when conducting focus groups and interviews, as well as gathering data via portfolios.

Interviews

Individual interviews provide one method of data collection that involves open-ended questioning. These in-depth conversations allow educators to elicit rich descriptions and explore issues. When conducting interviews, faculty should carefully construct the questions that will guide data collection. To enhance the conversation, the interview should be conducted in a mutually convenient private location and a relaxed atmosphere. With the availability of technology such as videoconferencing, interviews can now be easily conducted from a remote location. Many interviewers will use a semi-structured interview guide to direct key elements of the conversation, but prompts can help to probe for additional information. Interviewers may take notes during or after the session to aid recall of key aspects of the interview. Interviews can be audio-recorded followed by line-by-line transcription to provide a verbatim record of the interview for data analysis. Data analysis should yield common or reoccurring findings.

Focus Groups

Focus groups, another form of qualitative data collection, may be used for program evaluation. Essentially, focus groups consist of a guided conversation conducted by a trained facilitator who initiates an interactive conversation among participants. Using a carefully constructed interview guide and encouraging interaction, the facilitator elicits the sharing of ideas, feelings, attitudes, and opinions that leads to a collective understanding about the topic (Krueger & Casey, 2015; Ryan, Gandha, Culbertson & Carlson, 2014; Shaha, Wenzel & Hill, 2011). Box 6.6 provides some general guidelines for use of focus groups and some sample questions. The purpose of the focus group is not to reach consensus among the participants but rather to seek opinions and viewpoints. The facilitator creates an atmosphere that encourages interaction and a dynamic exchange that encourages conversation. Depending on the targeted group and topic, the exact size of the focus group may vary. In general, small groups of participants, usually five to eight, are recommended.

Faculty planning focus groups need to make a number of decisions about the data collection approach to ensure quality. They should carefully create open-ended questions that lead to conversational discussions. Planners also need to determine if they should provide the questions to the participants before the focus group to allow each respondent to consider the topic before data collection begins (Lewallen, 2015). Alternatively, they can choose to wait and use questioning only during the focus group session. Another factor that faculty need to consider involves sampling and recruitment of participants. Those participating in a focus group need to have experience or familiarity with the topic. For example, selecting first-semester students to engage in a focus group conversation involving their clinical experiences when they have participated in only a

---

BOX 6.6

Focus Group Guide and Sample Questions

Welcome the participants.

Explain the purpose and structure of the focus group.

Ensure privacy and confidentiality of the conversation.

Begin with an opening question or statement that can be answered by all and engages all participants, for example: Tell us your name and what program track you are enrolled in.

Ask key questions, for example:
    What do you think of _____?
    What do you like best about _____?
    What do you like least about _____?
    How has the program helped you to develop _____?
    How could the program be improved?
    Think back to _____ experience. What was that experience like for you?

Allow participants to offer differing points of view or confirm what has already been said.

Use pauses to allow participation.

Probe for additional information by using statements such as:
    Can you give an example?
    Would you explain what you mean by _____?

Conclude the group by asking about any missing information and thank participants.

---

few days of clinical learning would not provide ample conversations. Conversely, inviting senior students who have participated in numerous clinical learning opportunities to participate in a focus group to discuss their clinical experiences would lead to a much richer and descriptive conversation.

The identification and selection of participants is another important issue for consideration that can impact data collection and quality. A challenge that many focus group planners encounter involves scheduling and coordination of the focus group (Shaha, Wenzel, & Hill, 2011). Faculty should consider the pool of participants and their schedule demands and plan for focus groups that are conveniently scheduled, such as close to students' class time. Or, if planning a focus group for alumni, faculty should consider when potential participants would be available, such as during a time when alumni return to the school of nursing.

Unlike questionnaires that can be completed quickly, focus groups require more time for participation. Therefore, faculty should consider offering incentives to encourage participation. Depending on the budget and purchasing restrictions, small tokens of appreciation can be provided, such as bookstore or coffee shop gift cards, school supplies, and food. When carefully planned and executed, focus groups can provide valuable data that can assist with nursing program evaluation.

Portfolios

Many undergraduate and graduate nursing programs use portfolios to showcase student knowledge, skills, and achievements. They also can assist in evaluating the achievement of program outcomes (Haverkamp & Vogt, 2015; Karlowicz, 2010). Traditionally, educational portfolios were a collection of paper-based student works such as student papers, concept maps, journals, and evaluation materials. The materials were assembled to document growth, offer an opportunity for reflection, and assist with professional development (McDonald, 2014). With changes in student demographics, advances in technology, and the need for portfolio portability and accessibility of portfolio materials for faculty review, many nursing programs have shifted to an electronic or e-portfolio (Chertoff, 2015; Green, Wyllie, & Jackson, 2014; Haverkamp & Vogt, 2015; Willmarth-Stec & Beery, 2015). The purpose of the e-portfolio is the same as a traditional portfolio; however, diverse multimedia materials such as video, audio, and other digital artifacts can be included. Regardless of the format used for the portfolio, nursing programs continue to use them for assessment of program outcomes, but caution should be exercised to ensure that the methods of assessment are appropriate and yield meaningful data.

Faculty face a number of challenges when using portfolios for nursing program evaluation. One challenge is the time needed for creation, orientation, and evaluation of portfolio materials. To be used effectively, faculty need to commit time to provide feedback to students to assist them in professional growth. Students need orientation to the portfolio requirements and clear directions that guide portfolio creation. Faculty need to be clear about the purpose of the portfolio and determine if it will contain a collection of best works or be a growth-and-development portfolio that provides evidence of work in progress (Green, Wyllie, & Jackson, 2014). Additionally, careful construction of precise evaluation methods, such as scoring rubrics, and comprehensive and intensive evaluator training is needed. Karlowicz (2010) indicated that rubrics are used frequently for portfolio evaluation, but the measure and methods vary and issues related to reliability and validity are not clearly reported in the literature. She suggested use of a portfolio evaluation scoring tool, which has been tested to establish reliability and validity. Portfolio ratings are dependent on the type of portfolio entries, use of scoring rubrics, and evaluator training (Gadbury-Amyot, Krust, & Austin, 2014).

Existing Assessment Tools

Assessments made at the end of a program of study, sometimes referred to as exit examinations or exit evaluations, provide valuable assessment information that can guide program decisions. Faculty may feel overwhelmed in creating a survey that gathers comprehensive end-of-program information. They may face difficulty creating assessments that yield meaningful data and decide to use existing data collection tools rather than creating their own tool.

There are a number of existing assessment tools that are available for faculty to use for collecting nursing program evaluation data. Nationally or commercially developed tools offer a number of advantages. They are typically designed by test construction leaders who have access to significant resources, are tested with a broad sample of participants in diverse settings, and offer comparison data for programs.

One such existing assessment tool is offered by SkyFactor Benchworks, previously known as Educational Benchmarking Incorporated (EBI) (SkyFactor Benchworks, 2015). Assessment surveys developed by SkyFactor Benchworks gather data from graduating students, alumni, and employers. These standardized assessments can be used for program improvement and to assist with accreditation review activities. The surveys were created in collaboration with the American Association of Colleges of Nursing (AACN) and are aligned with the Commission on Collegiate Nursing Education (CCNE) accreditation standards (AACN, 2015). Due to their alignment with CCNE accreditation standards, many schools may find it easy to use such surveys to gather data and support accreditation self-study reports. Companies such as Skyfactor Benchworks offering these assessments provide programs with a comparative analysis of the data. Schools can compare their results with all test takers, self-selected similar schools, and institutions from similar Carnegie classifications (Diefenbeck, Hayes, Wade, & Herrman, 2011).

Other companies provide standardized surveys for data collection from students and alumni. Certified Background, a CastleBranch Corporation brand already used by many nursing programs for screening and compliance management, offers web-based surveys that may assist with nursing program evaluation (CastleBranch, 2012). Their products include a nursing student questionnaire that gathers information about student demographics, education, and employment. Additionally, they offer a postgraduate questionnaire that gathers contact information, program reflection, continuing education, and employment information from alumni. Nursing programs can add supplemental questions to the existing surveys and select timing for distribution, thereby providing for tracking of longitudinal data from nursing cohorts.

Regardless of the company or surveys selected, nursing programs need to carefully review these products, determine their alignment with the program outcomes, and evaluate how successfully the products fulfill data collection and program evaluation needs. Faculty need to consider student demographics, costs, availability, and delivery of products when making a decision to use existing tools.

CAPTURING DATA FROM KEY STAKEHOLDERS

Program evaluation plans typically include data collection from a variety of key stakeholders. Obviously, a major stakeholder is the nursing student. Many data collection strategies will involve soliciting student input and feedback throughout the program. Accessing and gathering data from students is not usually difficult, as they are easily accessible and frequently willing to provide the needed information. It also is important that data come from other key stakeholders including graduates and those employed in clinical agencies (preceptors, supervisors, and employers); however, gathering data from these groups can be challenging. There are some innovative approaches that can be used to enhance response rates and participant engagement with the data collection process.

In addition to the traditional strategies used to enhance the quality of data, faculty may consider some supplementary approaches that may assist with gaining access to key stakeholders and enhance responses. Many schools use advisory groups to provide input about the program and assist with strategic visioning and planning. Holding meetings at convenient, neutral locations may be helpful. Given demands such as travel time, parking availability, and cost, advisory meetings could be held at a location other than the nursing program. Faculty should consider neutral sites such as professional conferences and nursing meetings, at health care agencies, or in a private room in a public meeting space (Lewallen, 2015). Incentives such as a reception that includes food will make the environment welcoming and relaxed. Linking activities with well-attended existing campus, community, and professional events also may be helpful.

Technology Use

Emerging technology provides creative data collection opportunities. Social media use continues to grow, and online social networking sites such as Facebook and Twitter have experienced rapid growth. Facebook reports 968 million daily users (Facebook, 2015). It is the most popular social media website for college students, with estimates of between 85% and 99% of college students using this website to connect with others (Junco, 2012). Given the widespread use of social media, nurse educators may want to consider how this technology can be harnessed to enhance data collection and increase program evaluation responses. Some educators have reported success with technology-based data collection strategies. Story, Butts, Bishop, Green, Johnson, and Mattison (2010) experienced difficulty obtaining alumni responses using traditional mailed survey methods. In an effort to improve responses, they used Facebook to create a nursing program alumni group. A message was posted in the alumni Facebook group, which requested survey participation. This led to a dramatic increase in completed surveys, with responses going from almost zero to over 50% (Story et al., 2010).

Professional networking sites, such as Nurses Lounge (www.nurseslounge.com), also provide the opportunity for nursing programs to connect with students and alumni through onsite groups and announcements. Similar to Facebook, these professional nursing networking sites allow faculty in nursing programs to communicate with members. Other professional social networking sites, such as LinkedIn, also hold great potential for nursing program evaluation. Twitter, another popular application, provides an additional method for reaching alumni who may not respond to traditional survey methods. However, using Twitter has limitations as a program evaluation tool since it allows only short, 140-character messages or "tweets" that can be posted to the networking site (Bristol, 2013). Using social networking is a creative approach that provides an inexpensive and efficient method for reaching alumni. Many alumni are probably already engaged in social networking activities such as Facebook and Twitter.

Faculty considering using this approach for data collection need to realize the limitations of the technology for program evaluation. Only those with access to social media sites can be reached using these electronic methods. It is reasonable to assume that not all alumni are represented on social media. Additionally, faculty need the technology expertise to set up profiles, groups, and post messages using these networking websites. Faculty engaging in social media activities who do not have the knowledge and skills to use this data collection approach may need to enlist the support of others who are technologically savvy and familiar with these applications.

Developing technology also can be used to interact with clinical partners who are located at remote sites or who are unable to travel to campus to provide input for nursing program evaluation. Since faculty may have difficulty gathering data from clinical partners due to time demands, scheduling constraints, distance, and costs, alternative evaluation activities may be needed. Online programs, in particular, may find it difficult to evaluate program outcomes and may seek feedback from distant-site clinical partners. A variety of telecommunication videoconferencing options may assist in connecting with these key program stakeholders. Products such as Skype (www.skype.com), Zoom (http://zoom.us), Google Hangouts (https://hangouts.google.com/), Facetime (http://www.apple.com/mac/facetime/), and others allow users to capitalize on technology for videoconferencing, screen sharing of materials, sending files, or group calling. Online video chat programs allow for virtual meetings and interviews, and may have conferencing capabilities. Some of these communication platforms offer recording options to document a record of the videoconference session. Before implementing this approach for data collection, it is important to carefully select the platform that will be most effective, be available, and meet program and participant needs. Faculty should practice with the equipment and become familiar with the program before using it for formal data collection. Costs also need to be considered. Some video-conferencing programs are free while others that offer deluxe options or special features have a cost. Ease of use, quality of the audio and video, and the need for special equipment such as a webcam are other factors to consider. Lastly, faculty should evaluate if recording the session is needed. If a record of the videoconference is essential, then other factors to consider as part of the planning process are the Internet connection speed, computer technology compatibility, and preferred technology platforms.

ENSURING STANDARDS IN PROGRAM ASSESSMENT AND EVALUATION

Regardless of the tools used and data collection delivery method employed, faculty need to follow professional and ethical practices to ensure quality data and protect participants. The Joint Committee on Standards for Educational Evaluation (JCSEE, 2015) and Association for Institutional Research (AIR, 2013) provide educators with professional practice guidelines and program evaluation standards. These guiding documents provide useful information about integrity, responsibility, accountability, propriety, competence, confidentiality, utility, accuracy, and feasibility as they relate to program evaluation. Appendix B provides the JCSEE program evaluation standard statements that can be helpful in guiding program evaluation activities.

One important aspect of collecting program evaluation data that faculty need to consider involves confidentiality of information. It is critical for faculty to take measures to protect student information gathered as part of program evaluation and ensure confidentiality of participants. Sensitive information should be stored in secure locations. If electronic data are collected, it should require a password to access, and firewalls should be established to prevent unauthorized access. If data are collected via a website, a Secure Socket Layer (SSL) protocol will encrypt user data, thus offering an additional layer of protection (Fink, 2015). Since interviewers and moderators of focus groups will know the identity of participants, care should be taken to ensure confidentiality of data and protection of participant identity. Recording of pseudonyms or code numbers rather than names is one strategy that can be used to de-identify participants and enhance protection. Faculty reviewing and reporting data need to take measures to aggregate information and report group data.

The nursing program should establish guidelines or procedures for the use and access of all evaluation data. Collected data and participant information should be kept in locked filing cabinets or electronic files on secure password-protected computer drives. Program or institutional policies should direct when collected personal identifying information would be released to those with a legitimate educational or professional interest. Faculty must adhere to all applicable privacy laws such as the Family Educational Rights and Privacy Act (American Educational Research Association, American Psychological Association, & National Council on Measurement in Education, 2014; Shellenbarger & Perez-Stearns, 2010). Programs also should discuss how long they will retain evaluation data. Another consideration presented in national testing standards involves test security and protection of test copyrights. If using existing data collection tools, faculty need to obtain copyright permission and comply with administration guidelines and use of these items, including ensuring security of materials (American Educational Research Association et al., 2014).

Faculty involved with evaluative student data collection may want to consider review and approval by the Institutional Review Board (IRB) for the protection of human subjects before beginning data collection. Generally, if the faculty intend on sharing data gathered as part of program evaluation publicly for scholarly purposes, such as in professional presentations, publications, and reports, then the evaluation is considered research and thus needs IRB approval (Banta & Palomba, 2015; Fink, 2015, p. 243; Heflin, DeMeo, Nagler, & Hockenberry, 2015). These reviews may be expedited or considered exempt because there is minimal risk and may be part of normal educational practices. Since guidelines and standards for reviews can vary and change over time, it is always advisable to consult program and institutional policies and local IRBs to ensure that guidelines are followed. Regardless if a formal IRB proposal is required, faculty should adhere to the same ethical principles of beneficence, respect, and justice when collecting data for program evaluation purposes. Participation should be voluntary and not onerous, the benefits of participation should outweigh the risks, participants' identity should remain confidential, and data should be protected.

When conducting program evaluation activities it is important to prevent bias and ensure that uniform assessment approaches are used. Faculty should take steps to promote nondiscriminatory inclusive sampling and objective reporting. Data collection steps and analysis of the results should be transparent and clear for reviewers. Box 6.7 provides some suggestions for materials to include when documenting data collection activities.

BOX 6.7

Documentation of Data Collection

Participants
  Description of population
  Selection of participants, including criteria for inclusion or exclusion
  Representativeness of sample
  Characteristics of participants
Methods
  Context of data collection (methods to minimize distractions, standardize administration, maximize accessibility and fair testing, and minimize negative consequences)
  Protocols followed
  Tools used
  Timing of assessment
  Methods to establish reliability and validity
  Maintenance of integrity
  Data analysis techniques

SUMMARY

Program evaluation is a complex process involving many decisions. Faculty need to consider data sources, psychometric issues, and other factors that can impact quality. Decisions about the type of data needed and best tools to use to collect data are critical considerations. Determining how to capture data from key stakeholders while ensuring adherence to appropriate standards are also part of the choices that faculty make as part of the assessment and evaluation of nursing programs. Making good choices about the data collection process can lead to quality evaluation data that serve as the basis for well-informed, data-driven decisions for nursing programs.

References

American Association of Colleges of Nursing. (2015). *EBI assessment surveys*. Retrieved from http://www.aacn.nche.edu/research-data/ebi

American Educational Research Association, American Psychological Association, & National Council on Measurement in Education. (2014). *Standards for educational and psychological testing*. Washington, DC: American Educational Research Association.

Association for Institutional Research. (2013). *Code of ethics and professional practice (Code)*. Retrieved from http://admin.airweb.org/Membership/Pages/CodeOfEthics.aspx

Banta, T. W., & Palomba, C. A. (2015). *Assessment essentials: Planning, implementing, and improving assessment in higher education*. San Francisco, CA: Jossey-Bass.

Ben-Nun, P. (2008). Respondent fatigue. In Paul J. Lavrakas (Ed.), *Encyclopedia of survey research methods* (pp. 743–744). Thousand Oaks, CA: Sage.

Bristol, T. (2013). Accreditation management with technology. *Teaching and Learning*

in Nursing, 8, 36–39. doi: 10.1016/j.teln.
2012.10.001

CastleBranch (2012). *Future Focus*. Retrieved
from http://go.castlebranch.com/l/15312/
2015-03-06/2g7jjh

Chertoff, J. (2015). Global differences in
electronic portfolio utilization—a review
of the literature and research implications. *Journal of Educational Evaluation for
Health Professionals, 12*, 1–7. doi: 10.3325/
jeehp.2015.12.15

Diefenbeck, C. A., Hayes, E. R., Wade, G. H.,
& Herrman, J. W. (2011). Student-centered
outcomes evaluation of the clinical immersion program: Five years later. *Journal
of Nursing Education, 50*, 628–634. doi:
10.3928/01484834-20112729-02

Dillman, D. A., Smyth, J. D., & Christian, L.
M. (2014). *Internet, mail, and mixed-mode
surveys: The tailored design method* (4th
ed.). Hoboken, NJ: John Wiley & Sons.

Eder, D. J. (2014). Healthy assessment: What
nursing schools can teach us about effective
assessment of student learning. *Assessment
Update, 26*(3), 3–13. doi:10.1002/au

Facebook. (2015). *Our Mission*. Retrieved
from http://newsroom.fb.com/company-
info/

Fink, A. (2015). *Evaluation fundamentals:
Insights into program effectiveness, quality,
and value*. Thousand Oaks, CA: Sage.

Furr, M. F., & Bacharach, V. R. (2014). *Psycho-
metrics: An introduction*. Thousand Oaks,
CA: Sage.

Gadbury-Amyot, C. C., Krust, K., & Austin,
K. J. (2014). Fifteen years of portfolio assess-
ment of dental hygiene student competency:
Lessons learned. *The Journal of Dental
Hygiene, 88*, 267–274.

Green, J., Wyllie, A., & Jackson, D. (2014).
Electronic portfolios in nursing education:
A review of the literature. *Nurse Education
in Practice, 14*(1), 4–8. doi:10.1016/j.nepr.
2013.08.011

Haverkamp, J. J., & Vogt, M. (2015). Beyond
academic evidence: Innovative uses of technology within e-portfolios in a Doctor of
Nursing Practice program. *Journal of Professional Nursing, 31*, 284–289. doi: 10.1016/j.
profnurs.2015.03.007

Heflin, M. T., DeMeo, S., Nagler, A., &
Hockenberry, M.J. (2015). Health professions education research and the IRB.
Nurse Educator. http://journals.lww.
com/nurseeducatoronline/Citation/
publishahead/Health_Professions_Educa-
tion_Research_and_the.99860.aspx#. doi:
10.1097/NNE.0000000000000230

Horne, E. M., & Sandman, L. R. (2012). Current trends in systematic program evaluation of online graduate nursing education:
An integrative literature review. *Journal
of Nursing Education, 51*, 570–576. doi:
10.3928/01484834-20120820-06

Joint Committee on Standards for Educational
Evaluation. (2015). *Program evaluation
standards statements*. Retrieved from
http://www.jcsee.org/program-evaluation-
standards-statements

Junco, R. (2012). The relationship between
frequency of Facebook use, participation in
Facebook activities, and student engagement. *Computers & Education, 58*, 162–171.
doi: 10.1016/j.compedu.2011.08.004

Karlowicz, K. A. (2010). Development and
testing of a portfolio evaluation scoring tool.
Journal of Nursing Education, 49, 78–86.

Krueger, R. A., & Casey, M. A. (2015). *Focus
groups: A practical guide for applied research*.
Thousand Oaks, CA: Sage.

Lewallen, L. P. (2015). Practical strategies for
nursing education program evaluation.
Journal of Professional Nursing, 31, 133–140.
doi:10.1016/j.profnurs.2014.09.002

McDonald, M. E. (2014). *The nurse educator's
guide to assessing learning outcomes*.
Burlington, MA: Jones & Bartlett.

Oermann, M. H., & Gaberson, K. B. (2014).
Evaluation and testing in nursing education.
New York, NY: Springer.

Pallant, J. (2013). *SPSS survival manual: A
step by step guide to data analysis using IBM
SPSS*. Berkshire, England: Open University
Press.

Polit, D. F., & Beck, C. T. (2012). *Nursing
research: Generating and assessing evidence
for nursing practice*. Philadelphia, PA: Wolters
Kluwer/Lippincott Williams & Wilkins.

Ryan, K. E., Gandha, T., Culbertson, M. J., &
Carlson, C. (2014). Focus group evidence:

Implications for design and analysis. *American Journal of Evaluation, 35*, 328–345. doi: 10.1177/1098214013508300

Sauter, M. K., Gillespie, N. N., & Knepp, A. (2012). Education program evaluation. In D. M. Billings & J. A. Halstead (Eds.), *Teaching in nursing: A guide for faculty* (pp. 503–549). St. Louis, MO: Elsevier.

Shaha, M., Wenzel, J., & Hill, E. E. (2011). Planning and conducting focus group research with nurses. *Nurse Researcher, 18*(2), 77–87. doi: 10.7748/nr2011.01.18.2.78.c8286

Shellenbarger, T., & Perez-Stearns, C. (2010). From the classroom to clinical: A Family Educational Rights and Privacy Act primer for the nurse educator. *Teaching and Learning in Nursing, 5*, 164–168. doi: 10.1016/j.teln.2010.05.002

Skyfactor Benchworks (2015). *Assessment and benchmarking for nursing education programs, made easy*. Springfield, MO: Author.

Story, L., Butts, J. B., Bishop, S. B., Green, L., Johnson, K., & Mattison, H. (2010). Innovative strategies for nursing education program evaluation. *Journal of Nursing Education*, (49)6, 351–354. doi: 10.3928101484834-20100217-07

Sue, V. M., & Ritter, L. A. (2012). *Conducting online surveys*. Los Angeles, CA: Sage.

Willmarth-Stec, M., & Beery, T. (2015). Operationalizing the student electronic portfolio for doctoral nursing education. *Nurse Educator, 40*, 263–265. doi:10.1097/NNE.0000000000000161

7

The Accreditation Process in Nursing Education

Judith A. Halstead, PhD, RN, FAAN, ANEF

The quality of health care provided by the United States nursing workforce is largely dependent on the quality of the education in programs from which those nurses graduate. Accreditation is one public measure of quality assurance by which nursing programs can demonstrate quality to stakeholders of the educational process. This chapter describes the purpose of higher education (postsecondary) accreditation in the United States, types of accreditation, and the usual program elements represented in accreditation standards for nursing education. An overview of the accreditation process is also provided. The relationships among program evaluation, continuous quality improvement, and the accreditation process are emphasized.

PURPOSE OF ACCREDITATION

Accreditation of U.S. institutions and programs in higher education is a form of quality assurance and improvement, achieved through participation in an external quality review process. The overall purpose of accreditation is to protect the interests of the public. In the United States, accreditation has been in existence for over 100 years (Eaton, 2012a). Institutions and programs participate in the accreditation process as one means by which they can assure the students enrolled in their educational programs, as well as the general public, that they are offering quality education. The accreditation process is applied at the institutional level (colleges and universities) and the programmatic level (discipline-specific).

It is important to understand the distinctions between accreditation and regulatory authority, as they are different and independent processes (Kremer & Horton, 2016). For example, state boards of nursing are regulatory bodies that hold the authority to regulate both nursing practice and nursing education. Nursing programs cannot operate without state authorization to do so, granted to them by the appropriate state board of nursing. Some state boards of nursing term this authorization *approval* while other state boards of nursing use the term *accreditation*. Regardless of whether the term is approval or

---

BOX 7.1

Primary Roles of Accreditation

Serves as evidence of quality assurance to students and public
Grants institutions eligibility to access federal and state funding
Provides evidence of quality to community (employers, donors, among others)
Facilitates students' academic credit transfer between institutions

---

From Eaton, J. S. (2012a). *An overview of U. S. accreditation.* Washington, DC: Council for Higher Education Accreditation.

accreditation, the regulatory authorization granted by state boards of nursing is different from that of the accreditation status granted by national nursing accrediting agencies. Boards of nursing grant authorization for nursing programs to operate because they hold state regulatory responsibility for protecting the public's welfare, health, and safety (National Council of State Boards of Nursing [NCSBN], 2004). Nursing programs must be in compliance with the regulations set forth by the state board of the state (or states) within which they operate, or the board of nursing has the authority to suspend or close the operation of the program. In contrast, accreditation by a national nursing accrediting agency is a voluntary, nongovernmental process, which nursing programs opt to pursue as a public mark of quality assurance. While accrediting agencies can deny or revoke the accreditation of a program if the accreditation standards are not met by the program, they do not have the authority to suspend the operation of or close the program.

Historically, accreditation has been considered to be a voluntary activity that institutions and programs can choose to pursue. In reality, though, it is often an expectation for higher education entities to be accredited if they want to have access to federal and state funding for student financial aid and for programs of research and program development, as well as to benefit students in their search for postgraduation employment and further academic progression in their education. Recent actions by state legislators in a number of states also have made it mandatory for nursing programs to become accredited. Thus, while the accreditation process is described as voluntary, it is increasingly important that institutions and programs participate in the process.

The Council for Higher Education Accreditation (CHEA; Eaton, 2012a) described four primary roles for accreditation (Box 7.1). It is clear from these roles that stakeholders beyond the federal and state governments regard the accreditation status of the institution or program to be an important indicator of quality. In addition to the four primary roles identified by the CHEA, participating in the accreditation process requires the institution or program to formally engage in a systematic evaluation process, identifying strengths and areas for improvement and resulting in continuous quality improvement efforts.

ACCREDITATION AND ROLE OF THE U.S. DEPARTMENT OF EDUCATION

The U.S. Department of Education (USDE) is not directly involved in the accreditation of postsecondary institutions or programs. The role of the USDE in accreditation is to recognize accrediting agencies that are considered to be reliable authorities for setting standards and evaluating the quality of the institutions and programs that they accredit. As required by federal law, the USDE maintains a published national listing of all institutional and programmatic accrediting agencies recognized by the USDE (USDE, 2015a).

What is the USDE's vested interest in recognizing accrediting agencies? Postsecondary institutions and programs commonly seek federal funds to provide financial aid to students or to acquire grant funding for various institutional research and programmatic needs. As one eligibility criterion and measure of quality assurance, the federal government requires that institutions and programs applying for federal funding be accredited by a USDE-recognized accrediting agency, thus demonstrating that the institution or program has undergone an external peer review of the quality of its educational programming. The USDE is the federally designated department responsible for verifying the quality of the accrediting agencies that accredit U.S. institutions and programs. Seeking recognition from the USDE is a voluntary activity for accrediting agencies, and the USDE will recognize only those agencies that apply and meet criteria found in a published set of standards (USDE, 2015a).

Title IV and Accreditation

Some accrediting agencies are specifically recognized by the USDE to be "gatekeepers" of Title IV funds. Title IV of the Higher Education Act of 1965, amended, addresses the federal student financial assistance programs administered by the USDE. To be considered eligible for Title IV funding, institutions need to meet three criteria, known as the *program integrity triad:* (1) state authorization, (2) accreditation by a USDE-recognized accrediting agency, and (3) verification by the USDE of the institution's eligibility to manage federal financial aid programs (Skinner, 2007).

Therefore, it is required that any postsecondary institution or program wanting to administer federally funded financial assistance to its students be accredited by an accrediting agency that is recognized by the USDE for Title IV gatekeeping purposes. For the majority of postsecondary institutions and the academic programs that are housed within the institution, this requirement is met through accreditation by a regional or national institutional accreditor. However, in some cases, programs may be administratively housed in institutions that are not eligible for regional or national institutional accreditation. In nursing education, this most commonly happens in practical/vocational nursing programs and diploma nursing programs if they are located within technical institutions or hospitals. Such programs must then seek accreditation from a programmatic accreditor that is recognized by the USDE for Title IV purposes. In nursing, the only programmatic accreditor holding this recognition is the Accreditation Commission for Education in Nursing (ACEN).

TYPES OF ACCREDITATION

There are two types of accreditation in higher education: institutional and programmatic accreditation (USDE, 2015a). Institutional accreditation is awarded to all aspects of the entire college or university. Programmatic accreditation, also known as specialized accreditation, is granted to individual schools, programs, or departments, and is usually focused on a single discipline.

BOX 7.2

U.S. Regional Accrediting Agencies

Middle States Commission on Higher Education
New England Association of Schools and Colleges, Commission on Institutions of Higher Education
The Higher Learning Commission
Northwest Commission on Colleges and Universities
Southern Association of Colleges and Schools, Commission on Colleges
Western Association of Schools and Colleges, Accrediting Commission for Community and Junior Colleges
Western Association of Schools and Colleges, Senior Colleges and University Commission Colleges

---

Institutional Accrediting Agencies

Institutional accrediting agencies grant accreditation to colleges and universities. In 2011, there were 18 institutional accrediting agencies in the United States responsible for accrediting 7818 institutions (CHEA, 2011). There are three categories of institutional accrediting agencies: regional, national faith-based, and national career-related (Eaton, 2012a).

Regional accrediting agencies accredit private and public, two- and four-year degree-granting colleges and universities that are primarily nonprofit. There are seven regional accreditors, all of which are Title IV gatekeepers of federal funds (USDE, 2015b; Box 7.2). National faith-based accreditors, of which there are four, accredit institutions that have a religious affiliation and a mission that is primarily nonprofit and degree-granting. National career-related accrediting agencies accredit both degree-granting and nondegree-granting institutions that are predominately for profit and providing career-focused education. There are 12 national career-related accrediting agencies (Eaton, 2012b).

Achieving institutional accreditation benefits the institution's academic programs. The public mark of quality that institutional accreditation conveys is an assurance to the public that the institution has processes in place that enable it to meet established standards, maintain fiscal stability, employ qualified faculty, offer federally funded student financial assistance, have adequate student support services, and offer quality curricula. Having such solid institutional infrastructures in place, as indicated by achieving accreditation, assists programs in leveraging the resources of the institution to maintain their own quality and recruit students to their programs.

Programmatic Accreditation

As of 2011, there were 62 programmatic accreditors accrediting over 22,000 programs in the United States (CHEA, 2011). Academic programs such as nursing and other health professions, law, business, and engineering are examples of specific programs that are accredited by programmatic accreditors. These programs may be public or private, nonprofit or for profit.

Programs seek accreditation for several reasons. A primary reason is to demonstrate to the public that the quality of the education offered by the program meets established professional standards. Another reason is to use the accreditation standards to engage in continuous quality improvement efforts that will enhance the program's outcomes. Continuous quality improvement implies that the program has a systematic evaluation process in place that is ongoing and leads to databased improvement efforts. Accreditation may also qualify a program to seek federal and state funding to support research and programming initiatives, and also serves to benefit the program's students in future education and employment efforts. For example, in the nursing profession, many graduate nursing programs will not admit students who have not graduated from an accredited undergraduate program. Employers may also decline to hire nurses who have not graduated from accredited nursing programs, and some health care agencies will provide clinical learning experiences only for programs that are accredited.

In the nursing profession, there are three programmatic accrediting agencies that accredit nursing programs at large. Historically, the National League for Nursing (NLN) was the first nursing education program accreditor in the nursing profession, beginning accrediting activities in 1952. Currently, the NLN's accrediting activities are carried out by the Commission for Nursing Education Accreditation (CNEA). Established in 2013 as an autonomous accreditation division of the NLN, the CNEA accredits all types of nursing programs, including practical/vocational, diploma, associate, bachelor, master's and clinical doctorate programs. As a new accrediting agency, the NLN CNEA is in the process of seeking recognition by the USDE.

A second programmatic accreditor in nursing education is the Commission for Collegiate Nursing Education (CCNE). The CCNE is the autonomous accreditation arm of the American Association of the Colleges of Nursing (AACN). The CCNE accredits baccalaureate and higher-degree nursing programs and is recognized by the USDE.

The third programmatic accreditor in nursing education is the Accreditation Commission for Education in Nursing (ACEN), formerly known as the National League for Nursing Accrediting Commission (NLNAC). The ACEN accredits all types of nursing programs, and is the only nursing program accreditor recognized by the USDE as a Title IV gatekeeper for nursing programs that require this function of their programmatic accreditor.

There are also specialty accreditors in nursing education. The Council on Accreditation (COA) of Nurse Anesthesia is the accrediting agency for nursing programs that prepare nurse anesthetists. The Accreditation Commission for Midwifery Education (ACME) accredits nursing programs that educate nurse midwives. Both agencies are recognized by the USDE.

Nursing programs can select the nursing accrediting agency by which they wish to be accredited; some programs opt to be accredited by more than one agency. The program's administrators and faculty need to carefully consider which accreditation agency best aligns with the program's mission and goals before determining the agency that is the best fit for their program. While accreditation standards and policies can be similar, the values and philosophical approach to the accreditation process may vary among agencies.

ACCREDITATION STANDARDS

The accreditation standards that are promulgated by the accrediting agency form the focus of the accreditation process. Accreditation standards are applied at the institutional and program levels. At the program level, accreditation standards reflect the professional

---

BOX 7.3

Accreditation Standards Elements of U.S. Department of Education

Successful student achievement as related to institution/program mission, including course completion rates, licensure/certification rates, job placement rates
Curricula
Faculty
Facilities, equipment and supplies
Fiscal/administrative capacity
Student support services
Policies regarding advertising and publications (recruiting, admissions, grading, and so forth)
Description of program length and degree credentials*
Record of complaints received from students
Evidence of compliance with Title IV of the Higher Education Act*

---

*Expected of accrediting agencies recognized by the USDE for Title IV gatekeeping purposes. From U.S. Department of Education Office of Postsecondary Education Accreditation Division (2012). *Guidelines for preparing/reviewing petitions and compliance reports.* In accordance with 34 CFR Part 602 The Secretary's Recognition of Accrediting Agencies. Washington, DC: U.S. Department of Education.

standards, values, curricular concepts, and educational outcomes that are espoused by the profession. As such, accreditation standards are set by the profession itself and are inclusive of input from various stakeholders, such as educators, practice partners, and members of the public.

In addition to any accreditation elements that professions deem to be essential to ensuring quality in their specific educational programs, the USDE has identified some elements that USDE-recognized accrediting agencies are expected to include in their accreditation standards for institutions and programs. Box 7.3 provides a list of the elements of these expected standards. Because of these USDE expectations for recognized agencies, the accreditation standards of many accrediting agencies include a common set of standards and criteria, which are similar in nature and foci. Table 7.1 lists the areas of the accreditation standards for the ACEN, CCNE, and NLN CNEA. The USDE expectations for accreditation standards are described further in the following sections.

Successful Student Achievement

Accreditation standards are expected to address student achievement of program outcomes that are aligned with the institution's mission. Specific areas that need to be addressed include student success on licensure and certification examinations, program completion rates, and employment rates. It also is an expectation that programs will have an assessment and evaluation plan in place that fosters the collection and analysis of data

TABLE 7.1		
Accreditation Standards for ACEN, CCNE, and NLN CNEA		
ACEN	**CCNE**	**CNEA**
Standard 1—Mission and Administrative Capacity	Standard I—Program Quality: Mission and Governance	Standard I—Culture of Excellence: Program Outcomes
Standard 2—Faculty and Staff	Standard II—Program Quality: Institutional Commitment and Resources	Standard II—Culture of Integrity and Accountability: Mission, Governance, and Resources
Standard 3—Students		
Standard 4—Curriculum		Standard III—Culture of Excellence and Caring: Faculty
Standard 5—Resources	Standard III—Program Quality: Curriculum and Teaching/Learning Practices	Standard IV—Culture of Excellence and Caring: Students
Standard 6—Outcomes		
	Standard IV—Program Effectiveness: Assessment and Achievement of Program Outcomes	Standard V—Culture of Learning and Diversity: Curriculum and Evaluation Processes

ACEN, Accreditation Commission for Education in Nursing; CCNE, Commission for Collegiate Nursing Education; CNEA, Commission for Nursing Education Accreditation; NLN, National League for Nursing

designed to measure student achievement of expected outcomes, and will use the feedback from data analysis for purposes of program improvement (USDE, 2012, pp. 31–32).

Curricula

Standards related to program curricula are expected to address the specific degree level of the program and be correlated to the mission of the institution. The curricula of distance-education programs is expected to be similar to what is delivered on campus. In addition, standards are expected to address course sequencing, general education, and courses related to the major under study. Course objectives are expected to be clearly specified (USDE, 2012, p. 33).

Faculty

Faculty must have the requisite knowledge necessary to teach the courses to which they have been assigned and demonstrate the appropriate education and experience to qualify them for their teaching role. Standards are also expected to address the number of faculty required to adequately meet the program's mission. Criteria related to faculty development and evaluation are other key elements that are expected to be addressed in the standards (USDE, 2012, p. 34).

Facilities, Equipment, and Supplies

Demonstrating that the program has the resources necessary to achieve its mission and goals is an essential element of sustaining quality. The resources are inclusive of a budget that is sufficient to maintain and expand, as needed, the physical facilities for classrooms and laboratories; instructional equipment and supplies; and technical infrastructure that is sufficient to provide student support services and deliver distance education (USDE, 2012, p. 34).

Fiscal and Administrative Capacity

Expectations for this standard are that the program is able to demonstrate financial and administrative stability and there are adequate staff to implement the program's mission. It is important that program administrators have clearly defined roles and responsibilities and are qualified for their roles (USDE, 2012, p. 35).

Student Support Services

Standards related to student support services are expected to address the adequacy and effectiveness of the support services in helping students achieve academic success. Such support services may include having access to guidance related to financial aid, academic advising, career guidance, and personal counseling, among others. Maintaining the confidentiality of student records is another expectation (USDE, 2012, p. 36).

Policies about Advertising and Publications

Being accurate and clear in advertising and publications when communicating with program stakeholders is an important public demonstration of program integrity. The USDE expects that accrediting agencies will have standards that address the clarity and accuracy of the program's policies and practices related to recruiting and admissions, grading policies, and the publication of catalogs, academic calendars, recruitment materials, and other program documents (USDE, 2012, p. 36).

Description of Program Length and Degree Credentials

Accrediting agencies that serve as Title IV gatekeepers are expected to have standards that address usual program length and credit hours. This is aligned with their responsibility as a gatekeeper for student financial aid, as one means of ensuring that students are enrolled in programs that have curricula and required credit hours are congruent with program type and degree credentials. Programs not recognized for Title IV gatekeeping purposes are not required to address this element in their standards (USDE, 2012, p. 37).

Record of Complaints Received from Students

As one means of serving to protect student interests, it is an expectation that accrediting agencies will have standards that address student formal complaints and how they are managed by the program. It is an expectation that programs maintain records of student complaints, including documentation of how the complaints have been resolved (USDE, 2012, p. 38).

Evidence of Compliance with Title IV of Higher Education Act

In keeping with their responsibilities as Title IV gatekeepers, all accrediting agencies that have been recognized as such by the USDE are expected to have standards related to the institution's or program's compliance with Title IV regulations. Areas of compliance would include compliance audits, loan default rates, and other required reports as requested by the USDE (USDE, 2012, p. 38).

To summarize, accreditation standards are the foundation on which the accreditation process is based. Standards are developed by accrediting agencies and are derived from a profession's standards, values, curricular concepts, and expected educational outcomes. Additionally, the USDE has a set of standards expectations for all accrediting agencies that are recognized by the USDE. To achieve accreditation, institutions and programs must demonstrate their ability to meet the identified standards. They demonstrate their compliance by participating in the accreditation process, which is an external and public peer-review process.

THE ACCREDITATION PROCESS

"Accreditation is a standards-based, evidence-based, judgement-based, peer-based process" (Eaton, 2012b, p.14). Eaton's statement succinctly summarizes the accreditation process. Regardless of the agency conducting the accreditation process, certain elements will always be present. Those elements include a process that is focused on assessing the extent to which an institution or program meets a set of preestablished standards through the collection and analysis of data, and ultimately rendering a judgment (decision) by peers as to how successful the institution or program has been in demonstrating achievement of the standards.

When the nursing program is ready to begin the accreditation process, the initial step is to make contact with the selected accrediting agency, identify the types of programs seeking accreditation, and indicate the desire to start the formal steps of the accreditation process. The program will pay the accrediting agency a fee that will cover the costs associated with the accreditation site visit and other aspects of the process. The accrediting agency will provide the program with guidance on the typical timeline associated with the process; using this information, the program can best determine when to plan for an on-site program evaluation from the accrediting agency.

In the United States, the accreditation process consists of a series of steps designed to result in a comprehensive assessment and evaluation of the quality of the education provided by the program. The process allows for the program to engage in a self-assessment of program strengths and areas for improvement, as well as a peer review of the program. The decision-making body for the accrediting agency will consider evidence from both the program's self-assessment and peer-review process when rendering a decision regarding the accreditation status of the program. The steps that are usually associated with the accreditation process can be found in Box 7.4 and are discussed more fully in the following sections.

BOX 7.4

Steps of the Accreditation Process

1. Self-study: Process of program self-assessment
2. Peer review: On-site program evaluation visit
3. Accrediting agency judgment (decision)
4. Periodic review for continuing accreditation
5. Accreditation Reports

From Eaton, J. S. (2012a). *An overview of U.S. accreditation.* Washington, DC: Council for Higher Education Accreditation.

Self-Study: Process of Program Self-Assessment

The accreditation process always begins with the program administrators, faculty, and staff conducting a self-assessment of how they perceive the program to be meeting the accrediting agency's accreditation standards. Conducting such a process can take several months to complete, thus it is important for the program to plan accordingly and develop a timeline that allows enough time for the self-assessment to be completed in a reflective, thorough, and comprehensive manner. The outcomes of the self-assessment phase of the accreditation process are written in a narrative report that is commonly referred to as the "self-study." The self-study document is expected to address each accreditation standard and its criteria, providing data (evidence) of how the program is meeting the standard. In addition to the written narrative, documents that provide evidence of how the program is meeting the standards are included in the report's appendices.

Each accrediting agency has its own policies and procedures related to the format in which the self-study is to be written; the nursing program should carefully follow those guidelines. The length of the self-study will vary depending on the number of programs being addressed within the document. The self-study document is typically submitted to the accrediting agency six to eight weeks prior to the scheduled on-site program evaluation visit.

Peer Review: On-Site Program Evaluation Visit

Following submission of the program's self-study document, the next step in the accreditation process is to conduct an on-site evaluation visit by a team of peer evaluators. Peer evaluators are volunteers and not compensated for their services. The accrediting agency is responsible for appointing a team of evaluators, consisting of faculty and administrators from academia and nurses from practice. While the size of the team depends on the number of programs to be reviewed during the visit, it is most common to send a team of three or four program evaluators who are on-site for approximately three days.

It is the responsibility of the on-site program evaluation team to validate the data reported in the program's self-study document and seek any additional data needed to render a decision about the program's accreditation status. While visiting the nursing program, the team of evaluators reviews additional program documents and interviews a variety of stakeholders, such as faculty, institutional and program administrators, students, employers, and alumni. The on-site evaluators also visit clinical sites to observe students and faculty in the clinical learning environment.

At the conclusion of the visit, the on-site team conducts an exit interview with the program, summarizing the team's findings about the program's compliance with each of the accreditation standards. It should be noted that it is not the responsibility of the on-site team to formulate any recommendations regarding the program's accreditation status; accreditation decisions are the sole responsibility of the accrediting agency's board of commissioners (directors). Following the on-site visit, the visiting team of evaluators writes a team report that outlines its findings and submits the report to the accrediting agency. In turn, the accrediting agency provides a copy of the team report to the nursing program for review and response prior to forwarding the team report on to the agency's review committee. The nursing program is given the opportunity to correct any *factual data* errors that may be contained in the report. Following the program's review and opportunity to respond, as appropriate, the next step in the process is for the program's self-study and on-site evaluation team report to be forwarded to the accrediting agency's review committee.

Accrediting Agency Judgment (Decision)

On completion of the on-site evaluation visit, the next step in the accreditation process is to render a decision regarding the accreditation status of the program. The self-study document and on-site evaluation team's written report form the basis upon which the accreditation decision is made. While the process may differ depending on the agency, it remains a peer-review process. A common approach among nursing accrediting agencies is to forward the documentation to a review committee consisting of nurse educators and practice partners for consideration and to recommend a decision that is forwarded to the agency's board members for final action. Rendering the final accreditation decision is the responsibility of the agency's board, which is primarily composed of peers from education, as well as practice and public members.

The decisions that are rendered usually fall into one of three categories: (1) accreditation of the program, (2) accreditation of the program with conditions and progress report required, and (3) accreditation denied. In addition to the accreditation decision, the term of the accreditation is also granted. A program that is receiving initial accreditation will receive a shorter term of accreditation than programs being granted continuing accreditation. Depending on the nursing accrediting agency, an initial accreditation period is usually granted in the range of five to six years. For programs seeking a continuation of their accreditation status, an accreditation term of up to a maximum of eight years (ACEN) or 10 years (CCNE and NLN CNEA) may be granted.

All accreditation decisions are a matter of public record. The accreditation agency is required to publicly disseminate the outcomes of its review process and send notice to the USDE. Programs are also required to publicly disclose the outcomes of the review.

Periodic Review for Continuing Accreditation

After achieving initial accreditation, the program enters an accreditation cycle in which it will be reviewed for continuing accreditation at the designated time. The process for continuing accreditation includes the preparation of an updated self-study and another on-site evaluation visit. In between scheduled continuing accreditation visits, the program is required to pay annual fees and periodically send reports to the accrediting agency for review.

Accreditation Reports

Accredited programs have a responsibility to submit required reports to the accreditation agency on an annual basis. Such reports capture data related to student outcomes such as National Council Licensure Examination and certification pass rates; enrollment data; faculty numbers and qualifications; substantive changes in the program curricula, leadership, or financial status; and any other data that the accrediting agency deems important to ongoing monitoring of the program. Accrediting agencies evaluate the data and determine if there are any concerning changes in the program that may require a targeted visit to the program to gather additional information.

It is common for accrediting agencies to require a more extensive mid-cycle report from programs, in which they are asked to briefly address the accreditation standards and any changes that may have occurred since the last accreditation self-study and site visit. Through this reporting process, the program remains engaged in the continuous quality improvement process, and the accrediting agency is engaged in ongoing review of the program's outcomes.

SUMMARY

As a means of quality assurance and quality improvement, accreditation plays a significant role in shaping U.S. higher education. Similarly, accreditation significantly impacts the quality and outcomes achieved in nursing education. By embracing accreditation as a contributor to systematic program evaluation and using the outcomes of the process to engage in program improvement, nursing faculty are accepting the responsibility they have for providing students with quality education.

References

Council for Higher Education Accreditation. (2011). *CHEA almanac of external quality review.* Washington, DC: Council for Higher Education Accreditation.

Eaton, J. S. (2012a). *An overview of U.S. accreditation.* Washington, DC: Council for Higher Education Accreditation.

Eaton, J. S. (2012b). *Accreditation and recognition in the United States.* Washington, DC: Council for Higher Education Accreditation.

Kremer, M. J., & Horton, B. J. (2016). Accreditation of nursing programs. In D. Billings & J. Halstead (Eds.), *Teaching in nursing: A guide for faculty* (pp. 508–523). St. Louis: Elsevier.

National Council of State Boards of Nursing. (2004). *White paper of the state of the art of approval/accreditation processes in boards of nursing.* Chicago: Author. Retrieved from https://www.ncsbn.org/3954.htm

Skinner, R. (2007). Institutional eligibility for participation in Title IV student aid programs under the Higher Education Act: Background and reauthorization issues. CRS Report for Congress. Washington, DC: Congressional Research Service.

U.S. Department of Education (2015a). *Accreditation in the United States.* Washington, DC: US Department of Education. Retrieved from http://constructionlitmag.com/wp-content/uploads/2012/11/3169.pdf

U.S. Department of Education (2015b). *Regional and national institutional accrediting agencies.* Washington, DC: US Department of Education. Retrieved from http://www2.ed.gov/admins/finaid/accred/accreditation_pg6.html#RegionalInstitutional

U.S. Department of Education Office of Postsecondary Education Accreditation Division (2012). *Guidelines for preparing/reviewing petitions and compliance reports.* In accordance with 34 CFR Part 602 The Secretary's Recognition of Accrediting Agencies. Washington, DC: US Department of Education. Retrieved from http://www2.ed.gov/admins/finaid/accred/agency-guidelines.pdf

8

Program Evaluation:
Getting it Done in Your School of Nursing

Suzanne Marnocha, PhD, RN, CCRN, ret.
Jayalakshmi Jambunathan, PhD, RN

Accreditation is a vital process whereby schools/colleges of nursing meet identified standards. The process of accreditation is rigorous, holding schools to the highest standard of nursing education. Preparing for accreditation can be overwhelming. In this chapter, we offer some specific guidelines and helpful tips in preparing for the accreditation process in your school of nursing.

WHO SHOULD BE INVOLVED

All members of the school of nursing should be involved in the accreditation process. This is an opportunity for faculty, students, and staff to showcase with pride their school of nursing through the preliminary accreditation writing processes, building the resource base, designing an accreditation team room, and interacting with the accreditation team when they arrive. Since the accreditation process begins 18 to 24 months prior to the accreditation team site visit, roles and responsibilities of faculty and staff need to be defined early in the process. Writing groups should be formed for each of the accreditation standards and their respective criteria. The NLN Commission for Nursing Education Accreditation (NLN CNEA), Commission for Collegiate Nursing Education (CCNE), and Accreditation Commission for Education in Nursing (ACEN) standards were discussed in prior chapters. These groups should be led by a facilitator with prior accreditation experience. Faculty and staff participate in writing the self-study, adhering to a strict timeline with predetermined deadlines.

Our Process

In our school of nursing, the process began almost two years prior to the accreditation team site visit. A timeline was created to keep everyone on task, and deadlines were diligently adhered to. Writing groups were formed for each of the accreditation

---

BOX 8.1

Tips for Establishing Faculty and Staff Teams to Prepare Self-Study

Choose facilitators who have prior experience with the accreditation process.
Choose team members with the expertise required for each standard.
Create an 18- to 24-month timeline with specific deadlines.
Preassign staff for responsibility for each step in the accreditation process.
Post the timeline and schedule on your website for ease of access for all faculty and staff (this also allows everyone in the school to know the status of the accreditation process).
Assign one person to be responsible for the timeline and notification to groups as to their deadlines.
Create an atmosphere of group pride and responsibility.
Schedule regular update meetings.

---

standards and respective key elements. Each group was led by a senior faculty member or administrator who had been through the accreditation process previously. The dean and undergraduate program, graduate program, and research and evaluation directors served as group facilitators. Groups ranged from six to 10 members each and included a co-facilitator, faculty, and staff assigned based on their areas of expertise or interest. For example, the dean co-facilitated the standards related to mission, governance, and resources as she was the most knowledgeable about these areas; the largest number of faculty and academic staff worked on areas dealing with curriculum, teaching and learning, and student outcomes; and the director of research and evaluation facilitated the group related to evaluation processes and program effectiveness. Box 8.1 provides tips for assembling faculty and staff into groups to prepare the self-study.

SETTING UP PROCESSES FOR ACCREDITATION

It is important to start the planning process at least 18 months prior to the accreditation site visit. Planning may include a visit to the accreditation headquarters to review successful accreditation reports and collect pertinent information to make the accreditation process progress smoothly. Visiting websites of other schools of nursing to review their accreditation reports may be helpful in formatting your own report. Accreditation should be a standing agenda item at all appropriate committee meetings. Faculty, staff, and other stakeholders should be asked to participate in the accreditation process.

Our Process

When we started planning for accreditation, we discovered through the initial review that despite the copious collection of evaluation data, there was not a systematic review process. From this point on, our research director was the sole person responsible for conducting, analyzing, and reporting evaluation data through the nursing research office. Based on the research director's assessment of successful accreditation reports, an evaluation committee was established, with the research director as chair. Subsequently, the evaluation committee reviewed all evaluation data, with the nursing research office becoming the repository for all college of nursing evaluations. This also helped establish an easy retrieval system for any evaluation from all programs within the college. The evaluation committee began the process of analyzing five-year trends and establishing benchmarks, reviewing student satisfaction and alumni surveys related to outcomes, and examining data on student and employer satisfaction with the program—in essence, program effectiveness. Additionally, we visited websites to learn how to best format our accreditation report.

Simultaneously, other processes were taking shape in preparing for the site visit. Accreditation became a standing agenda item in all college of nursing meetings. At faculty meetings, faculty and staff were apprised of the purpose of the self-study and preparation process. Emphasis was on the importance of program effectiveness, outcomes, and how the self-study could help us bring about improvement relative to the changes that we had initiated. Accreditation group facilitators, along with their respective groups, presented on standard-specific progress. This proved to be a good venue for brainstorming. Most questions raised were answered by the group facilitator. However, in cases of ambiguity, detailed notes were taken, and clarification was sought through the official accreditation contact person at the accreditation office.

As the site visit drew nearer, one faculty meeting was devoted explicitly to the self-study report. This was held with the sole purpose of reflecting on and answering questions about the accreditation report, such as whether the narrative adequately addressed the standards, if it was clearly written, and if enough details and examples were provided to understand the process of self study used in the school.

Additionally, in our process, the dean's assistant was responsible for creating spreadsheets with specific timelines for each standard to facilitate clear expectations for the standards' groups to adhere to. Notification was given to nursing colleagues at our partner organizations of the impending accreditation dates and details, with the purpose of building a sense of community. The goal was to facilitate value and participation by all members of the community. These community-of-interest members included the Board of Visitors; university and college administrators; external stakeholders (hospitals, nursing homes, the local technical college); and other schools of nursing within our region.

Some strategies for setting up accreditation processes include:

- Visit websites to review accreditation report formatting.
- If possible, visit the accreditation headquarters to review successful accreditation reports and collect pertinent information to make the process go smoothly.
- Establish clearly defined roles and expectations for those involved in the accreditation process.
- Contact agency partners early to help them understand the accreditation process and obtain their support.

DATA COLLECTION

Data collection begins early in the accreditation process. Faculty, administrators, and others involved in accreditation should gather pertinent documents, both internal and external, related to each of the standards and respective key elements.

Our Process

Each of the standards groups was responsible for collecting data related to their specific standard, as well as checking all hyperlinks within their documents (nothing can be more frustrating for someone than to follow a link that goes nowhere). For example, the facilitator responsible for the standard related to evaluation contacted various departments for data related to program effectiveness: the nursing research office for evaluation data, alumni surveys, student and alumni satisfaction reports, and faculty outcomes; the graduate and undergraduate offices for enrollment data and trends, grievance reports, and certification pass rates from the previous three to five years; and the campus Office of Institutional Research for assistance with examining trends in student enrollments. With the assistance of these campus offices, we gathered all internal and external reports, which served as the foundation for the self-study report. Similarly, the curriculum standards group reviewed and analyzed the end-of-course responses by faculty and staff (Box 8.2).

BOX 8.2

End-of-Course Faculty Response

Course Number: Section: Semester:

Description:

1. Review goals and quantify data.
2. Summarize strengths, weaknesses, and suggestions for improvement or identified by the students.
3. Develop plan of action.
4. Download End-of-Course Faculty Report and complete.
5. Submit a typed written copy to the Undergraduate Program Office. Data for the Fall term are due by the 2nd Monday in March; Spring, by the 2nd Monday in November.

Section 1: Student Data

Course Strengths:
Course Weaknesses:

Section 2: Faculty Findings

Course Strengths:
Course Weaknesses:
Recommendations for course improvement (be specific and include dates for when):
Indicate the core competency in which you feel students displayed strengths:
Indicate the core competency in which you feel students displayed weaknesses:
Critique End-of-Course Evaluation tool used by students:

WRITING THE SELF-STUDY

The self-study report is an opportunity to involve many faculty and staff from the school of nursing to work as a team. The emphasis is to read each standard and key element carefully and capture enthusiastic points of pride along with data on accomplishments.

Our Process

As mentioned earlier in the chapter, we formed writing groups to increase faculty and staff involvement. Each standard and its criteria were facilitated by the director or the dean. Our goal was to "get it on paper" and then edit as necessary later. Box 8.3 provides tips for writing the self-study (Kremer & Horton, 2016).

We focused on analysis of data we had collected because this is critical to the success of the self-study, and it gave context and meaning to all evidence. We also submitted an electronic copy of the self-study document (including appendices), the program information form, agenda, and verification of the opportunity to selected stakeholders for their review and comments.

BOX 8.3

Tips for Writing Self-Study

1. Set timeline for completion of self-study and assign writing responsibilities.
2. Organize the self-study narrative according to standard and individual criteria.
3. Be cognizant of font requirements and page limitations.
4. Focus on providing a summary analysis with supporting documentation (evidence) of how standards and criteria are being met.
5. Provide documented examples of the program's data-based decision-making for each standard in narrative (with data sources available in on-site resource room or appendices):
   a. End-of-course reports
   b. Surveys and assessment of test results
   c. Committee minutes
   d. Evaluation summaries
   e. Outcome data
6. Use tables, graphs, and charts whenever possible to organize and present information.
7. Ensure each program and program option being addressed in the self-study, including distance education options, receives adequate attention in each standard.
8. In keeping with the process of continuous quality improvement, cite primary examples of the program's strengths, areas for improvement, and action plans for each standard.
9. Identify an individual who has final draft authority to comprehensively review document for accuracy, consistency, lack of duplication, adequate attention to each standard, and correct references to appendices and resource room documents.

Adapted from Kremer, M., & Horton, B. (2016) The accreditation process. In Billings, D. M., and Halstead, J. A. (Eds) *Teaching in nursing: A guide for faculty* (5th ed., pp. 508–523). St. Louis: Elsevier.

PREPARING FOR THE SITE VISIT

Faculty and administrators should plan for the site team visit at least six months in advance including planning for travel and accommodations, and getting to know the site team visitors. The school of nursing is responsible for paying for the flights, transportation, and hotel accommodations. The person assigned to pick up team members serves as the initial ambassador for *your* school and should be prepared to answer detailed questions about your school. It is important that all internal and external stakeholders recognize that each interaction is part of the site visit. Whoever is coordinating the site visit should inquire about specific needs of the team members, such as mobility. Housing should be at a comfortable and convenient location near the school, as the team members must be able to come and go without difficulty. In addition, the school should meticulously organize the document room (detailed in the next section) where evidentiary materials are stored.

Our Process

We started planning for the site team visit six months in advance by creating a step-by-step schedule, which included all of the on-site members and their specific duties (Appendix C, Table C.1). We made arrangements for each team member to be picked up at the airport at various times. We ensured that accommodations were comfortable and the location was close to the University for convenient visitor transportation. Since we were aware that the team would continue its work into the evening, we made sure that there was Internet access, a printer, and a meeting space large enough to accommodate a small group. In addition, we recommended that our faculty and staff learn the site team members' credentials ahead of time, for example, current role, clinical expertise, and research and publications.

DOCUMENT ROOM ORGANIZATION

For the document room, you should have an environment that allows the site team to easily locate and review necessary documents. It is important to create an index or resource room guide that directs the site visitors to where they can locate all materials. The physical work space should be well lit, quiet, and private. The work space should be a location that allows easy access to other resources in the school of nursing, including the main administrative offices and restrooms. The space does not have to be elaborate but should contain a large surface for reviewing materials. The document room is a visual display of materials to allow the team to understand how your nursing program meets their accreditation standards. Additionally, the room serves as a centralized location for the team to leave their belongings, review materials, and conduct executive sessions.

Our Process

We were particular with our document room organization. We selected a room that was well lit, quiet, and provided a large surface area for spreading out material and allow writing and keyboarding access (Figure 8.1). The physical space was large enough for

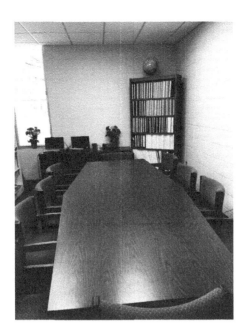

FIGURE 8.1 A resource room should be well lit and quiet, with a large desk. Copyright University of Wisconsin (UW) Oshkosh College of Nursing, Oshkosh, Wisconsin. Reprinted by permission of UW Oshkosh College of Nursing, Oshkosh, Wisconsin.

the team to accommodate their laptops and any documents for review. While we were cognizant that most evaluators travel with their own laptops, we provided laptops with Internet access and printers for the site team visitors. We created a resource room guide for the visitors to easily locate the materials that we had referenced in our self-study document (Appendix C, Table C.2). We had each of our evidence documents bound in hard copy in a file binder and also available electronically. We believe that this plan, although redundant, allowed for different preferences among the site team and eased their workflow.

We included the following documents in the resource room:

- Faculty curricula vitae consistently formatted to allow for ease of reading
- University reports: Copies of all pertinent reports were made available, including University accreditation documents, such as the Higher Learning Commission and all assessment and program reports.
- Minutes from all college of nursing committees
- Examples of student work
- College of nursing handbooks
- College of nursing bylaws
- Evaluation data and currently used forms, including student, alumni, employer, and other constituent survey instruments, and summaries/analyses of survey responses

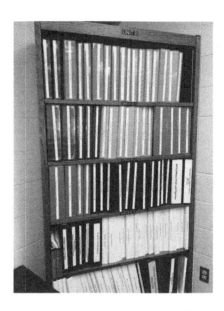

FIGURE 8.2 Resource room documents organization. Copyright University of Wisconsin (UW) Oshkosh College of Nursing, Oshkosh, Wisconsin. Reprinted by permission of UW Oshkosh College of Nursing, Oshkosh, Wisconsin.

We organized all documents in three-ring binders and color-coordinated each level and option of the undergraduate and graduate nursing programs (Figure 8.2). For example, the undergraduate program had blue binders organized with all syllabi located logically from front to back. Examples of class assignments and student work were placed within each binder to highlight successful attainment of university, program, and/or course outcomes. The self-study report selectively highlighted specific examples of individual courses and carefully cross-referenced meeting minutes, course syllabi, and student examples. We believed that it was important to cross-reference examples from our self-study document and have materials that easily followed with links to electronic and/or paper evidence. For example, if we discussed a curricular change, we documented where the initial idea originated (e.g., from national standards or research data, or feedback from students or community of interest), then tracked the progress of that idea through our own processes to final implementation and evaluation. Box 8.4 provides tips for planning the document room.

POTENTIAL PROBLEMS AND CHALLENGES

Problems may arise if the school is not prepared to address the questions from the team. You should have one person assigned to be the nursing program lead. This person is the primary contact for organizing the visit and may be the dean, director, chair, or another individual. You should plan ahead and have examples of materials that the team might ask for, for example, previous reports of NCLEX pass rates or copies of agency contracts. It is important to be clear about areas you might need to improve on and address them in the report.

BOX 8.4

Tips for Planning Document Room

Communicate preliminary planning details with only the team leader.

Assign one person to be in charge of all communication with the visiting team via the team leader, as well as for arranging transportation and accommodations for the accreditation team.

Arrange for transportation of team members from the first day they arrive until they leave.

Each communication is vital and may contribute to the report; select the correct person for each task.

Begin preparing the document room six months in advance.

Be organized and consider using three-ring binders that have clear labels and numbers on the outside of the binder edge for ease of location.

Have a clear index, with all pages numbered consistently.

Cross-reference documents by binder number and page.

Label documents consistently.

Make the process of finding examples easy for the team: for example, if you are discussing a change in course objectives, follow your own internal process, demonstrate the votes that occurred in each committee, and provide copies of the minutes and decisions. That way, the site reviewer can identify how you followed the proper process to discuss and approve curricular changes.

Provide both hard-copy and electronic documents.

Be certain that all links for online documents are current and active.

Provide office supplies, including a printer and paper for team use in the resource room.

Assign one person responsibility for all formatting and final submission.

Another possible area of concern is when your community of interest, including students, is not adequately prepared for the site visit. Students, agencies, and colleagues in the parent institution need to understand the purpose of the site team visit and how the school of nursing will be responding. You can send emails and letters to the community of interest explaining the accreditation process, their role, and dates of the site visit. It is important to point out the vital role for all members of the community in validating data and outcomes of the school of nursing. There should be one contact person in the school of nursing designated to reply to questions.

Students should be engaged six months in advance and taught about the terminology that the team might use, so that they can answer any questions honestly and clearly. One of our faculty members developed a unique idea to summarize our college visions, values, and mission and key terms. She developed a five-by-seven-inch "Accredit" card, printed on card stock, and distributed to all students, faculty, and staff, and shared with our Board of Visitors. When students met with the site visitors, they carried these and used them with pride. Nursing student leaders can become active members in preparing for the site visit and can teach other students about terms that the accreditation team might use and why the accreditation process is important.

SUMMARY

This chapter described the process of preparing for the accreditation site visit at our school. It is important that faculty and staff in schools of nursing work as a team at least 18 to 24 months prior to prepare for the site visit. Other strategies we used were provided in this chapter.

Reference

Kremer, M., & Horton, B. (2016), The accreditation process. In Billings, D. M., & Halstead, J. A. (Eds.). *Teaching in nursing: A guide for faculty* (5th ed., pp. 508–523). St. Louis: Elsevier.

9

Assessment of Online Courses and Programs

Karen H. Frith, PhD, RN, NEA-BC

Assessment of online courses and programs is an integral part of a nursing program's systematic program evaluation plan for continuous improvement and for accreditation. Regardless of the level of course or academic degree, guidelines and approaches have been developed that can promote effective assessment. This chapter addresses evaluating online courses, establishing benchmarks for program success, and assessing the quality of courses and programs using valid and reliable tools. Finally, the chapter describes the issues surrounding nursing courses and programs offered in other states as well as the impact on evaluation and accreditation.

EVALUATION IN AN ONLINE ENVIRONMENT

Accreditation

Nurse educators and administrators of online programs must ensure that resources are provided to support educationally sound courses that produce outcomes similar to courses offered on campus (Billings, Dickerson, Greenberg, Yow-Wu, & Talley, 2013). This premise reflects the standards for evaluation of online programs in nursing from regional accrediting organizations, such as the Middle States Commission on Higher Education and Southern Association of Schools and Colleges Commission on Colleges, and from nursing accreditation bodies including the National League for Nursing Commission for Nursing Education Accreditation (CNEA), the Accreditation Commission for Education in Nursing (ACEN), and the Commission on Collegiate Nursing Education (CCNE).

The Council of Regional Accrediting Commissions (C-RAC) developed the *Interregional Guidelines for the Evaluation of Distance Education,* also known as the C-RAC Guidelines (C-RAC, 2011). The C-RAC Guidelines include the following statements that should be used for evaluation of online education programs in nursing:

1. Online learning is appropriate to the institution's mission and purposes;

2. The institution's plans for developing, sustaining, and, if appropriate, expanding online learning offerings are integrated into its regular planning and evaluation processes;

3. Online learning is incorporated into the institution's systems of governance and academic oversight;

4. Curricula for the institution's online learning offerings are coherent, cohesive, and comparable in academic rigor to programs offered in traditional instructional formats;

5. The institution evaluates the effectiveness of its online learning offerings, including the extent to which the online learning goals are achieved, and uses the results of its evaluations to enhance the attainment of the goals;

6. Faculty responsible for delivering the online learning curricula and evaluating the students' success in achieving the online learning goals are appropriately qualified and effectively supported. The institution provides effective student and academic services to support students enrolled in online learning offerings;

7. The institution provides effective student and academic services to support students enrolled in online learning offerings;

8. The institution provides sufficient resources to support and, if appropriate, expand its online learning offerings; and

9. The institution ensures the integrity of its online offerings (National Council for State Authorization Reciprocity Agreements [NC-SARA], 2015a, pp. 11–12).

The C-RAC Guidelines contain additional information (action, processes, or facts) under each of the nine standards that institutions of higher education are to use to demonstrate the integrity of distance education programs (C-RAC, 2011). The entire C-RAC Guidelines can be found online at http://nc-sara.org/files/docs/C-RAC%20Guidelines.pdf.

The specialty accreditation organizations in nursing have accreditation standards that address online courses and programs. For example, the ACEN *Accreditation Manual Section III: Standards and Criteria* includes one criterion for each standard that addresses online education (ACEN, 2013). The CCNE *Standards for Accreditation of Baccalaureate and Graduate Nursing Programs* (2013) have no standards or key elements that are explicitly aimed at online education; instead, the requirement is that "all nursing programs seeking CCNE accreditation, including those with distance education offerings, are expected to meet the accreditation standards presented in this document. The standards are written as broad statements that embrace several areas of expected institutional performance" (CCNE, 2013, p. 2). Table 9.1 shows a comparison of distance education criteria in accreditation standards.

Accreditation in education typically focuses on governance, curriculum, resources, and achievement of learning outcomes. However, evaluation encompasses more than these broad components. Instructional design, interface usability, navigation of a course, and content design factors must all be evaluated (Wang, Solan, & Ghods, 2010). Without a well-designed course, students can spend too much time searching for content or assignments instead of achieving the intended learning outcomes.

TABLE 9.1

Comparison of C-RAC, ACEN, and CCNE Standards for Accreditation for Distance Education Programs

C-RAC Guidelines	ACEN Standards and Criteria	CCNE Standards and Key Elements
Online learning is appropriate to the institution's mission and purposes.	Distance education, when utilized, is congruent with the mission of the governing organization and the mission/philosophy of the nursing education unit.	No specific criteria for distance education
The institution's plans for developing, sustaining, and, if appropriate, expanding online-learning offerings are integrated into its regular planning and evaluation processes.	No specific criteria for distance education	No specific criteria for distance education
Online learning is incorporated into the institution's systems of governance and academic oversight.	No specific criteria for distance education	Faculty and students participate in program governance. Elaboration: Roles of the faculty and students in the governance of the program, including those involved in distance education, are clearly defined and promote participation. Nursing faculty are involved in the development, review, and revision of academic program policies.
Curricula for the institution's online-learning offerings are coherent, cohesive, and comparable in academic rigor to programs offered in traditional instructional formats.	Learning activities, instructional materials, and evaluation methods are appropriate for all delivery formats and consistent with the student learning outcomes.	The curriculum includes planned clinical practice experiences that: • enable students to integrate new knowledge and demonstrate attainment of program outcomes; and • are evaluated by faculty.

(continued)

TABLE 9.1		
Comparison of C-RAC, ACEN, and CCNE Standards for Accreditation for Distance Education Programs (*Continued*)		
C-RAC Guidelines	**ACEN Standards and Criteria**	**CCNE Standards and Key Elements**
		Elaboration: To prepare students for a practice profession, each track in each degree program and postgraduate APRN certificate program affords students the opportunity to develop professional competencies in practice settings aligned to the educational preparation. Clinical practice experiences are provided for students in all programs, including those with distance-education offerings. Clinical practice experiences involve activities that are designed to ensure that students are competent to enter nursing practice at the level indicated by the degree/certificate program. The design, implementation, and evaluation of clinical practice experiences are aligned to student and program outcomes.
The institution evaluates the effectiveness of its online-learning offerings, including the extent to which the online-learning goals are achieved, and uses the results of its evaluations to enhance the attainment of the goals.	Evaluation findings are aggregated and trended by program option, location, and date of completion and are sufficient to inform program decision-making for the maintenance and improvement of the student-learning outcomes and program outcomes.	No specific criteria for distance education

TABLE 9.1

Comparison of C-RAC, ACEN, and CCNE Standards for Accreditation for Distance Education Programs (*Continued*)

C-RAC Guidelines	ACEN Standards and Criteria	CCNE Standards and Key Elements
Faculty responsible for delivering the online-learning curricula and evaluating the students' success in achieving the online-learning goals are appropriately qualified and effectively supported.	Faculty (full- and part-time) engage in ongoing development and receive support for instructional and distance technologies.	Teaching-learning practices and environments support the achievement of expected student outcomes. Elaboration: Teaching-learning practices and environments (classroom, clinical, laboratory, simulation, and distance education) support achievement of expected individual student outcomes identified in course, unit, and/or level objectives.
The institution provides effective student and academic services to support students enrolled in online-learning offerings.	Orientation to technology is provided, and technological support is available to students. Information related to technology requirements and policies specific to distance education are accurate, clear, consistent, and accessible.	Academic support services are sufficient to ensure quality and are evaluated on a regular basis to meet program and student needs. Elaboration: Academic support services (e.g., library, technology, distance-education support, research support, admission, and advising services) are adequate for students and faculty to meet program requirements and to achieve the mission, goals, and expected program outcomes. There is a defined process for regular review of the adequacy of the program's academic support services. Review of academic support services occurs and improvements are made as appropriate.

(*continued*)

	TABLE 9.1	
Comparison of C-RAC, ACEN, and CCNE Standards for Accreditation for Distance Education Programs (Continued)		
C-RAC Guidelines	**ACEN Standards and Criteria**	**CCNE Standards and Key Elements**
The institution provides sufficient resources to support and, if appropriate, expand its online-learning offerings.	Fiscal, physical, technological, and learning resources are sufficient to meet the needs of the faculty and students to engage in alternative methods of delivery.	No specific criteria for distance education
The institution ensures the integrity of its online offerings (NC-SARA, 2015a, pp. 11–12).	No specific criteria for distance education	No specific criteria for distance education

ACEN, Accreditation Commission for Education in Nursing. CCNE, Commission on Collegiate Nursing Education. C-RAC, Council of Regional Accrediting Commissions.

Instructional Design

The design of online courses and teaching/learning approaches should be a concern for any nursing program. Standard 4 in the C-RAC Guidelines suggests that online course design and delivery methods (course management system) should enable and enhance the communication and active participation of students with each other and with their faculty members (C-RAC, 2011). A widely used tool for evaluating the overall course design is the *Quality Matters Higher Education Rubric* (Quality Matters, 2014). Faculty can engage in peer evaluation using the rubric or request review by the Quality Matters peer review team. Evaluation using the Quality Matters Rubric focuses on the alignment of elements of the course with each other to achieve desired student outcomes.

Interface Design

The design of the interface concerns the usability of the learning management system or other online technologies to minimize the cognitive load on students, making the system effective, efficient, and satisfying for students (The International Organization for Standardization [ISO], 1998). Even though faculty do not design their learning management systems, they are often asked to serve on a product selection committee. Knowledge of usability can assist faculty in the evaluation and selection of a learning management system that is user friendly for students and faculty.

Navigation Design

Faculty and instructional designers have control over the design of navigation within a learning management system. Most learning management systems are flexible enough to allow faculty to organize their courses in different ways; however, this flexibility can create a barrier to learning if navigation is different from course to course in an online program. Faculty involved in an online program should evaluate the navigation design across all courses in the program. If navigation is different, then faculty, in collaboration with instructional designers, can develop navigation templates for their online courses to standardize them.

Content Design

Faculty are content experts in the courses they teach, but they may need consultation with instructional designers to improve the online delivery of content to students. Innovations in technology and the adoption of technologies into online course offerings can be overwhelming to faculty who must keep current in nursing practice and scholarship. However, instructional designers who are up-to-date on the adoption of new technologies for pedagogical reasons make excellent partners for faculty content experts. For example, a faculty member teaching a course on evidence-based practice (EBP) could use an EBP model to organize the content and provide textbook and articles for students to read to learn the material. However, the content could be designed using synchronous video conferencing, asynchronous discussion boards, games, and other methods to increase interactivity and communication. Likewise, assignments can be completed in collaborative groups so that students learn together and from each other to achieve learning goals while increasing a sense of connection to each other.

Formative Evaluation

Evaluation should be designed into every online course. As students move through the content, data about student performance at the course level can automatically be generated through quizzes, discussion forums, polls, and other methods. Formative assessments should not be graded but rather used as a method of providing feedback to students as they are learning (Sewell, Frith, & Colvin, 2010). As with any formative evaluation, the data can be used to provide clarification about misunderstood concepts or to guide students to a deeper understanding. In addition, formative evaluation can be used to take corrective action in the design of the course during its delivery or prior to the next offering.

Summative Evaluation

Evaluation at the end of any course is performed to assess student learning outcomes (Billings et al., 2013) and student satisfaction with the course and faculty (Dae Shik, Lee, & Skellenger, 2012). Research has shown consistently that students who take online courses perform as well and sometimes slightly better than students in campus-based courses (Billings et al.). The evidence is clear that online education is a mainstream method for educating individuals in nursing programs when attention is given to the course design (Hoffmann & Dudjak, 2012), plan for communication and interaction of students and faculty (Avery, Cohen, & Walker, 2008), and preparation of faculty to teach using technology (Goodfellow, Zungolo, Lockhart, Turk, & Dean, 2014). Other summative evaluation appropriate to online courses can include technical assistance for students and faculty, support for diverse learning styles, and evaluation of faculty who teach in online courses (Avery et al., 2008; Goodfellow et al., 2014).

Formative and summative evaluation are of little value unless the data are used to adjust instruction or to make improvements in future course offerings. Therefore, formative and summative data from online courses, the actions taken by faculty, and resulting outcomes serve as complete cycles of improvement. Documentation of improvements can be saved for accreditation and presented to a curriculum committee to stimulate improvements across an online program.

ASSESSING QUALITY OF COURSES AND PROGRAMS

A closely related concept to summative evaluation is assessing quality of online courses and programs. Whereas summative evaluation focuses on the performance of students in a course and their satisfaction with that course, assessing quality of online courses and programs is a formal process for the measurement of indicators, use of the data to develop an improvement plan, and reassessment of the indicators to determine effectiveness. A nursing program might fold the online assessment plan into comprehensive assessment plans for on-campus programs or set them apart. In either case, nurse educators and program administrators work together to design an assessment plan that leads to continuous improvement and data-driven decision making.

There are several widely used frameworks for assessing quality in online education including the Western Interstate Commission for Higher Education's *Principles of Good Practice,* Online Learning Consortium (formerly Sloan-C) *Quality Framework,* and *Quality Matters* (Billings et al., 2013). Shelton (2011) identified and described 10 additional frameworks that can be used to assess quality in online courses and programs. Billings developed the *Framework for Assessing Outcomes and Practices in Web-Based Courses in Nursing* (2000); it has been widely cited in the literature. Billings' framework includes the assessment of technology, faculty support, student support, and educational practices outlined in the *Seven Principles for Good Practices in Undergraduate Education* (Chickering & Gamson, 1987) as factors leading to positive outcomes including learning. She identified outcomes relevant for online courses as recruitment, retention, and graduation; access; convenience; connectedness; preparation for real-world work; computer tool proficiency; professional practice socialization; and satisfaction (Billings, 2000, p. 61).

A nursing program can adapt a framework for assessing quality in online courses and programs by selecting representative indicators from each part of a framework. Once the framework and indicators are selected, the quality improvement plan can include indicators, benchmarks, data sources, persons responsible for assessment, frequency of assessment, actual outcomes, action plan, and action result. The plan then guides faculty and administrators to be deliberate in their approach to quality improvement.

Benchmarks for Program Success

Benchmarks are the expected outcomes that are set by faculty and administrators, which indicate that the program is successful. Nursing programs might set benchmarks based on the outcomes identified in the *Framework for Assessing Outcomes and Practices in Web-Based Courses in Nursing* (Billings, 2000). For example, nursing programs might select retention (also called persistence) and graduation rates as important outcomes because persistence has been a problem reported in the online education literature (Shea & Bidjerano, 2014). The faculty and administrators would need to set the benchmarks as desired or expected outcomes for their program. If the actual outcome falls short of the benchmark, the faculty and administrators would take action and reassess the indicator. Table 9.2 provides an improvement plan with a benchmark of 90% persistence in online courses and a benchmark of 80% graduation in an online program. Other benchmarks important to online programs include student engagement, satisfaction, and access to college or university resources. The following section on tools provides measurement of these more difficult indicators to quantify.

Tools

Nursing programs often use college- or university-developed tools to measure progress toward benchmarks for an entire online program. As an internal measurement, these tools work well if they are used to trend performance over time. However, faculty in nursing programs offering online courses who wish to compare their programs to similar programs or to conduct research can use published tools with established validity and reliability.

There are published tools that measure a philosophical approach to online education. The Community of Inquiry Framework (Garrison, Anderson, & Archer, 2001) focuses on three presences in online education: teaching, social, and cognitive presence. Arbaugh et al. (2008) developed the Community of Inquiry Instrument, which is a valid and reliable tool to measure the three presences. The tool contains 34 items, and factor analysis using principal components analysis and oblique rotation yielded three subscales. The subscales were found to be reliable with internal consistency (Cronbach's alpha) of 0.94 in the teaching presence subscale, 0.91 in the social presence subscale, and 0.95 in the cognitive presence subscale (Arbaugh et al., 2008).

Nursing programs that use a constructivist pedagogy stress learning as an interaction with existing knowledge and creation of new knowledge through engagement. Programs with such a focus might use the National Survey of Student Engagement (NSSE) to examine engagement (Meyer, 2014). The NSSE does not focus on online education per se, but reports on 10 engagement indicators important to online education including academic challenge, learning with peers, experiences with faculty, and campus environment (Center for Postsecondary Research, 2015). The items are scored on a 0 to 60 scale with answer options of never (0 points), sometimes (20 points), often (40 points), and very often (60 points). A mean is calculated in each of the 4 engagement categories and then weighted based on demographics in the sample. The validity and reliability of the NSSE is extensively documented at http://nsse.indiana.edu/html/psychometric_portfolio.cfm.

Nursing programs that use the *Seven Principles of Good Practices in Undergraduate Programs* (Chickering & Gamson, 1987) as the framework for their online programs could use a survey created by Crews, Wilkinson, and Neill (2015). The survey contains 36 items with Likert-type answer options. All items are matched to the seven principles. The authors of the survey did not offer any reliability assessments, but the tool has face validity. The survey could easily be adapted for use in nursing programs.

TABLE 9.2

Sample Plan for Measuring Quality in Distance Education Courses and Programs

Assessment Indictor	Benchmark for Success	Data Sources	Responsible	Schedule	Location of Document	Actual Outcomes	Action Plan	Action Result
Persistence in MSN online courses	90% of students registered for an online course complete the course.	Information system for student records	Adviser, Program Director, Curriculum Committee	At the end of each semester	Table of Quality Measurements reported in the Curriculum Committee Minutes	85% of students in fall semester completed online courses. 10% of students never logged into the learning management system (LMS) across all courses.	The Curriculum Committee voted to require orientation at the beginning of each semester for all online courses. Faculty agreed to send a list of students who had not logged into the LMS after the first 3 days of the semester to the adviser for follow-up.	In spring semester, 92% of students completed courses with only 3% never having logged into the LMS. Recommend: Continue monitoring and adviser follow-up.
Graduation rates in the MSN online program	80% of students enrolled in the online MSN program complete the program in 8 semesters.	Information system for student records and MSN database	Adviser, Program Director, Curriculum Committee	Yearly after graduation	Table of Quality Measurements reported in the Curriculum Committee Minutes	78% of students who enrolled in the first MSN online course completed the online program.	The Adviser and Program Director will use an early warning system to track continued registration of students who start the online MSN program. Students who have not registered within 2 weeks of the start of registration will be contacted by email or telephone.	The follow-up with students at registration revealed that most students who had not registered were waiting until financial aid was available. The Program Director will work with Financial Aid and the Registrar to look for solutions. Recommend: Continue monitoring with early warning system.

ONLINE PROGRAMS OFFERED IN OTHER STATES AND IMPACT ON EVALUATION AND ACCREDITATION

State Authorization

State governments have the authority to authorize higher education degrees or courses offered within their boundaries. The approval process includes degrees and courses offered on-campus as well as degrees and courses offered through online technologies. The United States Department of Education (USDOE) published regulations in October 2010 regarding state authorization of postsecondary education through distance education (Western Cooperative for Educational Technologies, 2014). The final regulations (Chapter 34, § 600.9(c)) required an institution offering postsecondary education through distance or correspondence education to meet state requirements. In addition, the institution has to document this to the Secretary of State's approval (USDOE, 2011). The regulation was later dropped in 2012, meaning that the deadline for complying with the federal regulation would not be enforced, but institutions of higher education would still be responsible for authorization by states.

The cost of state authorization on institutions of higher education that offer online courses and degrees is high. Personnel are hired to monitor conflicting, changing state laws and regulations and to seek approvals from state governments. Fees charged by state governments vary, making institutional planning difficult (Commission on the Regulation of Postsecondary Distance Education, 2013). The process of state authorization is slow and can require multiple submissions and visits to the state agencies to discuss the institution's educational offerings (National Council on State Boards of Nursing [NCSBN], 2014). With the growth of online courses and programs, state governments have been faced with requests from hundreds of institutions across the 50 states (NCSBN, 2014).

These aforementioned problems have been difficult for both higher education institutions and state governments. In response to the problems associated with state authorization, the four regional education compacts (Midwestern Higher Education Compact, New England Board of Higher Education, Southern Regional Education Board, and Western Interstate Commission for Higher Education) established a cooperative agreement called the State Authorization Reciprocity Agreement (NC-SARA, 2015a). One of the purposes of the SARA is to make state authorization more efficient and less burdensome on institutions of higher education and on states. Other purposes of the SARA include giving guidance on accreditation and institutional quality to avoid redundancy in accreditation requirements, providing a means for consumer protection, and defining institutional financial responsibility to avoid additional regulations for online education (NC-SARA, 2015a). The newly released *SARA Policies and Standards* require the chief executive of institutions to attest to compliance with the *Interregional Guidelines for the Evaluation of Distance Education* (described earlier in the chapter).

States interested in enrollment in the SARA must first be members of a regional education compact. Once a member, the state can enroll in the SARA. The enrollment process began in January 2014; as of this writing, there were 29 states in the SARA (NC-SARA, 2015b). For more information about the SARA, readers should visit the National Council for State Authorization Reciprocity Agreements to review the frequently asked questions document found at http://www.nc-sara.org/files/docs/SARA-FAQs.pdf.

Even though the SARA provides a more consistent and streamlined approach to state authorization for institutions in member states, institutions of higher education with nursing programs have additional requirements because of regulations by state boards of nursing (NC-SARA, 2015a). Institutions that offer online courses or degree programs leading to professional licensure are required to keep prospective students informed about the program's status with regard to state licensing requirements by providing such information in writing. If the institution cannot confirm whether the course or degree meets requirements for professional licensure in a prospective student's state, the institution is required to provide the student with current contact information for the state board of nursing in which the student lives (NC-SARA, 2015a).

National Council of State Boards of Nursing

The NCSBN issued a white paper on nursing regulation of distance education, which provides background information about online education, definitions, and general guidance for state boards of nursing. Two key definitions for the general guidelines are home and host state/jurisdictions. The home state/jurisdiction is "where the distance education program has legal domicile, and the host state/jurisdiction is the state/jurisdiction outside of the home state/jurisdiction where students participate in didactic coursework and/or clinical experiences" (NCSBN, 2015, p. 2). The NCSBN proposed the following guidelines for distance education prelicensure nursing education programs:

- Programs shall meet the same approval guidelines as any other prelicensure program in the home state;
- The home state/jurisdiction approves prelicensure nursing education programs, including distance-learning education programs;
- Programs in the home state provide oversight over the students in the host states and are responsible for the students' supervision;
- Faculty, preceptors, or others who teach clinical experiences for a prelicensure nursing education program by means of distance education should hold a current and active nursing license or privilege to practice, which is not encumbered, and meet licensure requirements in the state/jurisdiction where the patient is located. Faculty who teach didactic content for a prelicensure nursing education program by means of distance education shall hold a current and active nursing license or privilege to practice, which is not encumbered, and meet licensure requirements in the home state where the program is approved; and
- State Boards of Nursing will communicate information through their annual reports about prelicensure nursing program that have students enrolled in clinical experiences in host states (NCSBN, 2015, pp. 7–9).

The NCSBN's white paper provides a timeline for adopting the guidelines for distance education (NCSBN, 2014). The timeline includes the NCSBN and state boards of nursing responsibilities to adopt the guidelines as common requirements for prelicensure distance education across all states and jurisdictions by 2020. In the meantime, the NCSBN hosts a web page on prelicensure distance education requirements for the states and territories located at https://www.ncsbn.org/cps/rde/xchg/ncsbn/hs.xsl/671.htm (NCSBN, 2015). Some state boards of nursing require extensive approvals, while others have few requirements. For example, a nursing program with distance education offerings whose "home state" is Georgia could have a student living in and wanting clinical experiences in California (host state). In this case, the nursing program would check the NSCBN website and find that California's regulations state, "California-RN requires that only students enrolled in California-RN Board approved schools can participate in clinical experiences. Online out-of-state enrolled students would not be able to do clinicals in California-RN, unless the out-of-state program is California-RN Board approved" (NCSBN, 2015). If the student lived in and wanted clinical experiences in Virginia as the "host state," there are no regulations by the Virginia State Board of Nursing. The lack of common requirements for all state boards of nursing adds to the confusion and costs for nursing programs offering distance education (NCSBN, 2014).

Contracts for Clinical Affiliations

Because many state boards of nursing have not changed their regulations to match the guidelines from the NCSBN, nursing education programs offering online courses with clinical experiences must check the regulations for each state in which students plan to do their clinical experiences before sending clinical affiliation contracts to health care agencies in the host state. Even when a nursing program gets state board of nursing approvals, getting the host state health care agencies to sign clinical affiliation contracts usually takes months and may not be successful. Because of the long period of time to obtain a clinical affiliation contract, nursing programs should begin the process at admission or early in the student's enrollment in an online course or program.

SUMMARY

Assessment of online course and programs follows similar strategies used for campus-based education, including concern for accreditation and quality improvement. The assessment can be designed as a stand-alone process or integrated into a nursing program's comprehensive assessment plan. Faculty who teach and administrators who have programmatic responsibility for online courses and programs have added responsibility for compliance with regulatory requirements from host states and the boards of nursing. A systematic program evaluation plan that is based on a model for continuous improvement in online education can be a nursing program's best asset to maintain quality in all offerings.

References

Accreditation Commission for Education in Nursing (ACEN). (2013). *Accreditation Manual Section III: Standards and Criteria.* Retrieved from http://www.acenursing.net/manuals/SC2013.pdf

Arbaugh, J. B., Cleveland-Innes, M., Diaz, S. R., Garrison, D. R., Ice, P., Richardson, J. C., & Swan, K. P. (2008). Developing a community of inquiry instrument: Testing a measure of the Community of Inquiry framework using a multi-institutional sample. Part of a special section of the AERA Education and World Wide Web Special Interest Group (EdWeb/SIG), 11(3/4), 133–136. doi:10.1016/j.iheduc.2008.06.003

Avery, M. D., Cohen, B. A., & Walker, J. D. (2008). Evaluation of an online graduate nursing curriculum: examining standards of quality. *International Journal of Nursing Education Scholarship, 5*(1).

Billings, D. M. (2000). A framework for assessing outcomes and practices in Web-based courses in nursing. *Journal of Nursing Education, 39,* 60–67.

Billings, D. M., Dickerson, S., Greenberg, M., Yow-Wu, B., & Talley, B. (2013). Quality monitoring and accreditation in nursing distance education programs. In K. Frith & D. Clark (Eds.), *Distance education in nursing* (3rd ed.). New York: Springer Publishing Company.

Center for Postsecondary Research (2015). *National Survey of Student Engagement.* Indiana University School of Education. Retrieved from http://nsse.indiana.edu/html/about.cfm

Chickering A. W., & Gamson Z. F. (1987). Seven principles for good practices in undergraduate education. *American Association of Higher Education Bulletin, 39*(7), 3–6.

Commission on Collegiate Nursing Education (CCNE). (2013). *Standards for Accreditation of Baccalaureate and Graduate Nursing Programs.* Retrieved from http://www.aacn.nche.edu/ccne-accreditation/Standards-Amended-2013.pdf

Commission on the Regulation of Postsecondary Distance Education. (2013). *Advancing Access through Regulatory Reform: Findings, Principles, and Recommendations for the State Authorization Reciprocity Agreement (SARA).* Retrieved from http://nc-sara.org/files/docs/Commission-on-Regulation-of-Postsecondary-Distance-Education-Draft-Recommendations.pdf

Council of Regional Accrediting Commissions (C-RAC). (2011). *Interregional Guidelines for the Evaluation of Distance Education.* Retrieved from http://nc-sara.org/files/docs/C-RAC%20Guidelines.pdf

Crews, T., Wilkinson, K., & Neill, J. (2015). Principles for good practice in undergraduate education: effective online course design to assist students' success. *MERLOT Journal of Online Learning and Teaching, 11*(1), 87–103.

Dae Shik, K., Lee, H., & Skellenger, A. (2012). Comparison of levels of satisfaction with distance education and on-campus programs. *Journal of Visual Impairment & Blindness, 106,* 275–286.

Garrison, D. R., Anderson, T., & Archer, W. (2001). Critical thinking, cognitive presence, and computer conferencing in distance education. *American Journal of Distance Education, 15*(1), 7–23. doi:10.1080/08923640109527071

Goodfellow, L. M., Zungolo, E., Lockhart, J. S., Turk, M., & Dean, B. (2014). Successes and challenges of a distant faculty model. *Nursing Forum, 49,* 288–297. doi:10.1111/nuf.12060

Hoffmann, R. L., & Dudjak, L. A. (2012). From onsite to online: Lessons learned from faculty pioneers. *Journal of Professional Nursing, 28,* 255–258. doi:10.1016/j.profnurs.2011.11.015

International Organization for Standardization (ISO). (1998). Ergonomic requirements for office work with visual display terminals (VDTs) Part II: Guidance on usability. 9241-11:1998.

Meyer, K. A. (2014). Student engagement in online learning: What works and why. *ASHE Higher Education Report, 40*(6), 1–114. doi: 10.1002/aehe.20018

National Council for State Authorization Reciprocity Agreements (NC-SARA). (2015a). *SARA Policies and Standards.* Retrieved from http://www.nc-sara.org/files/docs/FINAL%20SARA%20General%20Policies%20released.pdf

National Council for State Authorization Reciprocity Agreements (NC-SARA). (2015b). *SARA States & Institutions.* Retrieved from http://nc-sara.org/sara-states-institutions

National Council on State Boards of Nursing (NCSBN). (2014). *Nursing Regulation*

Recommendations for Distance Education in Prelicensure Nursing Programs. Retrieved from Chicago, IL: https://www.ncsbn.org/cps/rde/xchg/ncsbn/hs.xsl/6662.htm

NCSBN. (2015). *Prelicensure Distance Education Requirements.* Retrieved from https://www.ncsbn.org/cps/rde/xchg/ncsbn/hs.xsl/671.htm

Quality Matters (2014). *The Quality Matters Higher Education Rubric* (5th Ed.). Retrieved from https://www.qualitymatters.org/rubric.

Sewell, J., Frith, K., & Colvin, M. (2010). Online assessment strategies: A primer. *MERLOT Journal of Online Learning and Teaching, 6.* 297–305. Retrieved from http://jolt.merlot.org/vol6no1/sewell_0310.pdf

Shea, P., & Bidjerano, T. (2014). Does online learning impede degree completion? A national study of community college students. *Computers & Education, 75,* 103–111.

Shelton, K. (2011). A review of paradigms for evaluating the quality of online education programs. *Online Journal of Distance Learning Administration, 4*(1). Retrieved from http://www.westga.edu/~distance/ojdla/spring141/shelton141.html

United States Department of Education (USDOE). (2011). *Code of Federal Regulations. Chapter VI—Office of Postsecondary Education, Department of Education. Chapter 34,* § 600.9(c). Retrieved from http://www.gpo.gov/fdsys/pkg/CFR-2011-title34-vol3/xml/CFR-2011-title34-vol3-subtitleB-chapVI.xml#seqnum600.9

Wang, J., Solan, D., & Ghods, A. (2010). Distance learning success—a perspective from socio-technical systems theory. *Behaviour & Information Technology, 29,* 321–329. doi:10.1080/01449290903544645

Western Cooperative for Educational Technologies (WCET). (2014). *State Approval of Out-of-State Providers.* Retrieved from http://wcet.wiche.edu/advance/state-approval-history

10

Evaluation of Specific Program Types and Impact on Program Assessment and Evaluation

Joan Such Lockhart, PhD, RN, CORLN, AOCN, CNE, FAAN, ANEF
Melinda G. Oberleitner, DNS, RN

As nursing program administrators scramble to meet societal needs for an ever-increasing supply of nurses at the entry and advanced-practice levels, they are often faced with the reality of administering multiple, disparate programs. For example, despite nursing programs often being labeled as "expensive" to offer, many schools of nursing offer an array of educational tracks and concentrations, including the following: programs targeted to prelicensure students with and without previous degrees; RN to Bachelor of Science in Nursing (RN to BSN) programs; RN to Master of Science in Nursing (MSN) programs; master's programs with multiple concentrations; post-master's degree offerings and certificate programs; and programs leading to terminal degrees such as BSN to Doctor of Nursing Practice (DNP), Doctor of Anesthesia Practice (DNAP/DrAP), DNP, and Doctor of Philosophy (PhD) programs. As the structure, resource requirements, and outcomes of academic programs are as unique as the graduate that the program is preparing, developing program assessment and evaluation plans with components relevant to each program is critical.

This chapter focuses on specific program types and their impact on program assessment and evaluation. Attention is paid to select programs to illustrate the need for unique assessment: (1) RN to BSN, (2) accelerated second career, (3) nurse practitioner, (4) nurse anesthetist, and (5) DNP and PhD programs. These areas are important to assess in addition to the typical components of program evaluation discussed in prior chapters.

RN TO BSN PROGRAMS

Almost 700 RN to BSN programs are in operation in the United States. More RN to BSN program options are available than are four-year nursing programs and accelerated baccalaureate nursing programs for nonnursing college graduates; approximately 60% of RN to BSN programs are delivered in online or hybrid formats (American Association of Colleges of Nursing [AACN], 2015b). Many schools offer accelerated programs in five-, seven-, or eight-week sessions with multiple start dates during the calendar year rather than longer, more traditional semester-based, fall, spring, and summer session offerings. Typical program completion times of students enrolled in RN to BSN programs is between one to two years.

The rapid proliferation of RN to BSN programs in response to national calls for increasing articulation opportunities for nonbaccalaureate graduates has spurred some concerns about program quality, academic rigor, and student progression and graduation rates, especially of students matriculating in online RN to BSN programs. To date, there are no national standards or guidelines from national nursing or professional organizations that provide direction for examining program effectiveness related to RN to BSN programs, as accrediting organizations typically evaluate RN to BSN programs within the context of the prelicensure BSN degree program, if one is offered by the school of nursing undergoing accreditation. In 2012, AACN released a white paper, *Expectations for Practice Experiences in the RN to Baccalaureate Curriculum* (AACN, 2012), in an effort to provide clarity to expectations of one aspect of RN to BSN programs—the need for quality practice experiences and opportunities for nurses enrolled in those programs.

Assessment and evaluation of student learning outcomes, although a major and primary component, is but one factor in program evaluation of RN to BSN programs. In the absence of national standards unique to RN to BSN program evaluation, assessment and evaluation of student achievement (including retention, progression, and graduation rates), curriculum relevance, and assessment of satisfaction measures should be undertaken with the ultimate goal of using ongoing and systematic evaluation to refine key processes and improve student learning.

Student Progression Tracking

Program assessment and evaluation aspects germane to RN to BSN programs include establishment of benchmarks related to student progression, attrition, retention, and graduation rates. Many schools also track persistence rates of students. However, there is lack of standardization in definition of these terms and of measurement processes, as well as an absence of national nursing standards related to tracking student progression (Robertson, Canary, Orr, Herberg, & Rutledge, 2010). For example, the National Center for Education Statistics Integrated Postsecondary Education Data System provides definitions for retention rates and graduation rates but not for attrition and persistence although retention is a measure of persistence. Typically, these rates are not tracked or measured by unique disciplines at the system or university level. To further complicate matters, some boards of nursing expect nursing schools to track graduation rates and may require their own methods of calculation (although many boards of nursing do not regulate postlicensure programs). Thus, it becomes incumbent on nursing faculty and administrators to define important terms and establish reliable term-to-term and year-to-year tracking and comparison methods.

Research indicates that RNs who return to school for their degrees are self-directed individuals who are willing to assume responsibility in achieving an important career goal. However, program flexibility, such as options to complete the program in online and accelerated formats, appear to be key components to degree completion (Matthews & Travis, 1994; O'Brien & Renner, 2000). Recently, Mancini, Ashwill, and Cipher (2015) conducted a comparative analysis of RN to BSN students (N = 3802) enrolled in on-campus and online RN to BSN programs at one university to better understand outcome variables in these populations. Although there were significant differences between the two groups, failure and drop-out rates for both groups were similar. The authors concluded that an online RN to BSN program, when designed using best practices for online education, has the potential to attain educational outcomes in this population that are similar to on-campus programs.

Curriculum

As stated earlier, there are no national guidelines or recommendations related specifically to the curricular structure of RN to BSN programs or to the unique end program competencies expected of their graduates. Hooper, McEwen, and Mancini (2013) presented recommendations for structuring RN to BSN programs. These included ensuring that RN to BSN students receive equal course credits as traditional prelicensure students in upper division nursing and nonnursing courses; requiring a full array of liberal arts courses; and providing course content that was focused directly on role differences of diploma/associate degree nurses and BSN nurses to encompass effective role-transition strategies. Some of this content may require clinical experiences in the RN to BSN program, comparable to experiences afforded to traditional students.

There appears to be considerable consensus in the literature as to which course content should be included in RN to BSN curricula (McEwen, White, Pullis, & Krawtz, 2014; Stokowski, 2011; Texas Board of Nursing, 2011; Wros, Wheeler, & Jones, 2011). This includes leadership/management, community/public health, nursing research/evidence-based practice, and professionalism/legal and ethical issues. In one study, program directors rated inclusion of problem solving/critical thinking and safety concepts as the most critical content to be included in RN to BSN curricula. The directors also rated high acuity, illness/disease management, infection control, and care transitions content as "somewhat important" or "not critical" in RN to BSN programs (McEwen et al., 2014). Absent any national guidelines related to essential curricular content in RN to BSN programs, these findings may inform content mapping for program assessment and evaluation purposes related to curricular structure.

Ensuring quality of curricula in RN to BSN programs offered in online formats presents additional program evaluation challenges. Well-recognized national organizations and programs that are committed to ensuring high quality in online course development and delivery include the Quality Matters (QM) program. The QM framework is one example of a faculty-centered peer-review process that can be used by online RN to BSN programs to certify the quality of courses offered in online and hybrid formats, and ensure adherence to best practices in online course delivery.

Program Satisfaction Indicators

Data related to satisfaction with specific aspects of the RN to BSN program can be collected in a variety of formats. In addition to data collected from student evaluations of teaching and other satisfaction surveys, interviews and focus groups of students, graduates, employers, and faculty can identify strengths and weaknesses of the program, including opinions of the academic rigor and reputation of the program, and can provide direction for program change, enhancement, and improvement. Focus groups have been successfully conducted in online programs using web-conferencing formats. Opinions and observations of individuals in auxiliary support capacities, such as library, tutoring, financial aid personnel, and faculty teaching in general education courses, can be important in identifying areas of concern and potential for improvement of the RN to BSN program.

ACCELERATED SECOND CAREER PROGRAMS

Accelerated second career (ASC) programs offer individuals who have completed undergraduate degrees in nonnursing fields the opportunity to complete their BSN degree in as few as 11 to 18 months (AACN, 2015a) or their MSN degree in three years (AACN, 2015a). ASC programs were originally developed by schools in an effort to increase their capacity and meet the career needs of nonnursing degree graduates who were interested in nursing (Fang, Bednash, & Dewitty, 2012). The rapid growth in ASC programs helps to alleviate the national nursing shortage by preparing qualified graduates who are ready to enter the nursing workforce in a short period of time. In addition, accelerated BSN (ABSN) programs address the Institute of Medicine's (IOM) recommendation to increase the number of BSN nurses to 80% by 2020 (IOM, 2010).

In the United States, ABSN programs have rapidly increased over the past 40 years. Nearly 300 programs were in operation by 2013, located throughout 46 states, the District of Columbia, and Puerto Rico, with 13 additional programs in progress (AACN, 2015a). Student enrollment and graduation rates from ASC programs also have grown, with 16,935 students enrolled in ABSN programs in 2014, an increase of 14 students from 2013 (AACN, 2015a). Growth has also been noted in fast-track options available for students completing their MSN (AACN, 2015a), with 62 accelerated or entry-level master's programs available in 2013 and nine programs under development (AACN, 2015a).

Accelerated programs must meet the same curriculum standards and accreditation criteria as their traditional BSN and MSN degree counterparts, and must produce competent graduates prepared to transition to clinical practice. The rapid pace of ABSN programs demands constant attention to assessment and program evaluation efforts with data supporting timely, evidence-based program improvement. While all components of program evaluation are important, ABSN programs, in particular, require attention to (1) curriculum and teaching-learning practices, (2) program outcomes, and (3) transition to practice.

Curriculum and Teaching-Learning Practices

Because ABSN programs target learners who have successfully completed a prior degree, faculty should design curricula that allow students to successfully attain expected learning outcomes in a short period of time. Innovative teaching-learning strategies that are tailored to adult learners and build on their past experiences should be integrated in all courses. Schools need to create a supportive environment that fosters effective learning and academic success.

The integration of adult-learning needs within a 15-month ABSN program was assessed using student focus groups that centered on their learning needs and program expectations (Robert, Pomarico, & Nolan, 2011). Focus groups were embedded in two courses at the beginning and end of the program. Data obtained at the first session were used by faculty to tailor their teaching strategies. Although program-end data reflected positive changes in teaching strategies and a collaborative interest in student success, students wanted additional attention to individual learning styles. Special attention to pedagogy for ABSN students was also suggested by Newton and Moore (2013), whose study revealed higher critical thinking skills among students in their accelerated program as compared with their traditional students at program entry.

Several qualitative studies that explored the experiences of faculty who teach in ABSN programs suggest a need to prepare both faculty and students for their respective roles. Using a hermeneutic phenomenology approach to explore the experiences of faculty teaching in ABSN programs, Cangelosi (2013) discovered that most of her 14 experienced and new faculty were unprepared to teach ABSN students, who often challenged them. The study theme of "Figuring It Out on My Own" (p. 277) conveyed faculty's need for role models and additional teaching support and guidance.

These findings mirror those reported by Brandt, Boellaard, and Zorn (2013), who also explored the experiences and emotions of 138 ABSN faculty from 25 randomly selected Midwestern programs. The study themes reflected a wide range of mixed emotions and experiences expressed by faculty, which included both frustration and satisfaction in teaching students who were highly motivated and diverse, and the large amount of work that was involved for both students and faculty. Results can be used for faculty development, support, and program improvement.

In another published report drawn from the same pool of participants (Boellaard, Brandt, & Zorn, 2015), faculty offered advice to other faculty interested in teaching ABSN programs. Their suggestions were embedded in study themes that included planning for program intensity, which is often stressful for both students and faculty; being available, flexible, open-minded, and patient; upholding established expectations and rigorous standards; preparing for challenging questions; knowing the material being taught; integrating students' diversity into teaching and learning approaches; and adapting content and teaching strategies to align with student and program characteristics (p. 343). Similarly, Driessnack et al. (2011) asked graduates (N = 8) from a Midwestern ABSN program to share examples of effective teaching strategies that they had experienced that met their learning needs. Themes included: "we are different; we feel overwhelmed with information; focus on teaching us process, not content; give us context; show us something new; group work does not equal team work; [and] the preceptors understand us" (p. 214).

Program Outcomes: Recruitment, Retention, and Predictors of Success

The rapid pace and intensive study involved in ABSN programs demand attention to recruiting applicants who can successfully complete program requirements in a timely manner, pass their licensure examination on the first attempt, and successfully transition into clinical practice. Collecting and analyzing program outcome data from key stakeholders such as the graduates themselves, employers, and faculty are essential to determine program effectiveness, foster continuous quality improvement (Commission on Collegiate Nursing Education [CCNE], 2013), and establish best practices for accelerated programs (Kemsley, McCausland, Feigenbaum, & Riegle, 2011). Nugent and LaRocco (2014) provided an example of an ABSN program review created retrospectively using input from graduates and faculty over an eight-year history. Results were used to shape changes in curriculum, teaching-learning practices, and costs. Kemsley et al. (2011) collected program feedback from ABSN alumni about their experiences from their preadmission period to graduation. Although these graduates rated the program highly, they offered insight into curriculum recommendations such as taking graduate-level courses and interfacing with graduate students while being ABSN students.

Program evaluation studies have also attempted to predict "success" among ABSN graduates using graduation and NCLEX-RN pass rates (Penprase & Harris, 2013; Steunkel, Nelson, Malloy, & Cohen, 2011). Payne, Glaspie, and Rosser (2014) compared ABSN outcome data with those collected from traditional BSN programs and found no significant differences in nursing GPA, NCLEX-RN® performance, Health Education Systems, Inc. (HESI™) examination scores, and pass rates between ABSN (n = 73) and traditional students (n = 189).

Transition to Practice

ABSN programs also require careful follow-up after graduation to evaluate the performance of graduates in their new professional roles. It is important to obtain the perspectives of key stakeholders such as employers, graduates, and faculty, and to compare these outcomes with graduates from traditional BSN programs. Employers' perspectives were reported by Rafferty and Lindell (2011) who found comparable results in the clinical competencies of ABSN and traditional BSN graduates as rated by their nurse managers. Ratings included six dimensions such as leadership, critical care, teaching/collaboration, planning/evaluation, interpersonal relations/communication, and professional development. Oermann, Poole-Dawkins, Alvarez, Foster, and O'Sullivan (2010) used focus groups to gather the perspectives of nurse managers about new graduates' performance. Managers reported that, although the maturity and experience helped ABSN graduates transition to clinical practice, both types of graduates were not clinically prepared for beginning nursing practice.

Self-reports were captured by Oermann, Alvarez, O'Sullivan, and Foster (2010), who found no difference between ABSN and traditional graduates related to performance, satisfaction, and transition to practice, despite a slight increase in mean performance ratings (excluding research) over their first year of employment. Similarly, Penprase (2012) investigated the perspectives of ABSN alumni about their transition into practice by asking them what influenced them to stay at the bedside and how faculty and employers can best prepare them for their transition. Respondents cited the value of preceptorships, orientation, and staff support among the most important factors that helped them transition. Using a different approach, Raines (2010) compared the ratings of nursing practice competencies from the perspectives of ABSN and unit-based experts from program start to end. Significant differences were noted between student self-ratings between the two time points and student and expert ratings; unit experts rated students higher than students rated themselves.

NURSE PRACTITIONER PROGRAMS

Nurse practitioners (NP) comprise a robust growth component of the health care workforce with over 200,000 NPs licensed in the United States today (American Association of Nurse Practitioners [AANP], 2015). To meet the growing demands for NPs and other advanced practice registered nurses (APRNs) in the United States, the number of programs preparing APRNs increased by 17% from 2010 through 2015. The largest APRN program growth, by far, has been in entry-level NP programs, in which enrollment grew by 81% in the same five-year period. As of fall 2013, 368 programs enrolled 56,496 students in master's NP programs, and 92 programs enrolled 5,064 students in post-BSN DNP NP programs. In comparison, during the same reporting period, 148 master's clinical nurse specialist programs enrolled 2,020 students, 40 master's nurse midwife programs enrolled 1,377 students, and 67 master's nurse anesthesia programs enrolled 3,532 students (AACN, 2015f). The demand for APRNs is projected to increase by over 30% through 2022, a growth rate that is faster than the average (11% growth) for other professions (Bureau of Labor Statistics, 2014).

Standards governing NP education include those relevant to all APRN roles established by professional organizations and accrediting bodies as well as standards specific to the NP role such as those explicated in the *Criteria for Quality Nurse Practitioner Education Programs* document (National Task Force on Quality Nurse Practitioner Education, 2012). Programs preparing NPs also must comply with expectations and requirements of the APRN Consensus Model (APRN Consensus Work Group and National Council of State Boards of Nursing APRN Advisory Committee, 2008).

Issues in the Clinical Education of NPs

Administrators are being forced to grapple with numerous challenges facing schools of nursing preparing NPs today. The most serious of these, with the potential to negatively impact programmatic outcomes, are a national shortage of qualified nursing faculty to meet enrollment demands, burgeoning student numbers, and growth in numbers of programs preparing NPs, which frequently leads to competition among schools for preceptors and quality clinical sites. Some schools of nursing are reporting pressure to provide compensation and incentives to preceptors and clinical sites in return for placing students at those sites.

The current model of clinical education for NPs has traditionally been an apprenticeship model with one preceptor overseeing the clinical performance of one student at a time. As program and student numbers continue to increase and as the expectations associated with NP and MD roles in practice become increasingly more complex, this model is rapidly becoming unsustainable in many areas of the country. To address these pressures and challenges, national nursing education organizations are calling on educational program administrators to pilot and evaluate outcomes of alternative models of APRN clinical education (AACN, 2015f).

Clinical education and evaluation models, which have been tested and validated in other health care professions, illustrate some potential feasible alternatives to traditional methods of clinical education and evaluation for NPs. For example, most accredited physical therapy (PT) educational programs in the United States and Canada voluntarily use standardized competencies and competency-based clinical assessments developed in collaboration with the American Physical Therapy Association. Preliminary work and discussions related to clinical instrument tool validation and use of a standardization tool in nurse anesthesia student clinical education has been initiated as well (Collins & Callahan, 2014).

Many of the same issues impacting programs providing NP education such as proliferation of mandated student assessment requirements, increased risks of losing clinical sites, and growing litigation and academic grievances related to lack of standardization in student assessment and evaluation practices precipitated efforts toward the creation of a standardized clinical evaluation instrument in PT. The Physical Therapy Clinical Performance Instrument (PT CPI) is used by academic educators and clinical preceptors. Although its use is voluntary, about 93% of accredited PT programs use the PT CPI for student performance assessment (Roach, Frost, Francis, Giles, & Nordrum, 2012).

Key elements related to use of the PT CPI include: (1) an annual registration fee paid by students, preceptors, and faculty is required to access the web-based system; (2) participation in standardized web-based training is mandatory prior to use of the tool by students, preceptors, and faculty to develop experience in rating student performance through case scenarios and practice questions; (3) preceptors complete the CPI on students and students complete self-assessments also using the CPI, documentation is available on the system throughout the clinical experience, and summative evaluations are conducted at mid-point and final evaluations; and (4) academic program and clinical coordinators have immediate access to performance assessment results as well as learning contracts, learning objectives, weekly planning forms, and critical incident reports. The web-based system facilitates retrieval and management of data including student and preceptor-related data. Aggregated data and reports are available to inform curricular change, to complete accreditation reports, and for research purposes (Frost, 2015).

Some alternative models for clinical teaching in graduate nursing programs currently being explored include dedicated education units (DEUs) in graduate education, which are being tested at the University of Pennsylvania through the Graduate Nursing Education Project; teaching the didactic contact in the beginning of the NP program with end-of-program clinical immersion experiences at the end; and increasing use of simulation. One of the goals of these models is to test the utility of moving from time-based advancement of students through the educational process to competency-based assessment and advancement. This shift could potentially help to alleviate many of the challenges faced by nursing programs in the clinical education of NPs and could result in greater opportunities for interprofessional practice experiences and shared competency-based student and programmatic assessments (AACN, 2015f; Frost, 2015).

NURSE ANESTHETIST PROGRAMS

Nurse anesthesia (NA) education in the United States is over 100 years old. As of late 2015, there were 113 accredited NA programs in the country (American Association of Nurse Anesthetists [AANA], 2015). These programs graduate approximately 2,000 students annually after the student has completed a minimum of seven calendar years of education and almost 2,500 clinical hours as part of the educational process. Currently,

37 NA programs have been approved to award the doctoral credential as entry into practice. The accreditation process for NA programs began in the early 1950s. The Council on Accreditation of Nurse Anesthesia Programs (COA) is the accrediting body for NA programs at the post-master's certificate, master's, and doctoral degree levels (COA, 2015). After 2015, the COA will no longer consider new master's degree programs for accreditation review. Beginning January 1, 2022, all students accepted into an accredited NA program must graduate with the doctoral degree.

One of the COA accreditation criteria under the Program of Study standard relates to student admission criteria. While the COA criteria delineate only two admission criteria, registration as an RN and at least one year of experience as an RN in a critical care area, many NA programs use other admission criteria. An issue of particular relevance in program evaluation of NA programs includes analysis of student admission criteria and the impact of those criteria on student progression.

Student Admission and Progression

Admission into NA programs is a highly competitive process. Typical admission criteria include assessment of the applicant's overall grade point average (GPA), GPA in science courses, scores on the Graduate Record Examination (GRE), and years of acute care experience, especially in critical care areas. However, what is the state of the evidence linking admission criteria other than those required by the COA to the NA applicant's ability to successfully integrate theory and practice, which results in positive progression to graduation?

Ortega, Burns, Hussey, Schmidt, and Austin (2013) conducted a systematic review to examine the evidence for evaluating applicants for admission into NA programs. Due to the limited number of sources and of the weak and dated available evidence, the authors determined there were no consensus factors that predict overall student success in NA programs. However, admission criteria with predictive value for success in the anesthesia program included overall GPA, science courses GPA, and nursing program GPA. GRE score was found to be less predictive in the studies reviewed. Length of time out of a formal education program was inversely related to success in the NA program. Similarly, in a study of four accredited NA programs to determine validity of clinical evaluation tools, preadmission overall GPA was found to have high predictive value in determining students' abilities to transfer didactic knowledge to the clinical setting, to troubleshoot equipment, and to perform technical skills related to practice, thus suggesting that overall GPA is an important preadmission criterion to retain in NA programs (Collins & Callahan, 2014). In related research, Burns (2011) conducted a quantitative correlational study of 914 anesthesia student records to determine if a relationship existed between admission criteria (overall GPA, GPA in science courses, GRE scores, and critical care experience) and academic progression in NA programs. The measures with the highest predictive value in this study were the overall preadmission GPA and GPA in science courses.

Finally, many NA programs use methods such as face-to-face interviews in an effort to capture information regarding applicants' noncognitive attributes including communication styles, interpersonal interactions, and leadership qualities. One interesting pilot study used high-fidelity simulation to evaluate applicants' cognitive and noncognitive attributes in addition to the traditional face-to-face interview (Penprase et al., 2012). A finding of this pilot was a positive correlation between scores on the simulation and face-to-face interview scores, suggesting that there may be a role for simulation in assessing cognitive and noncognitive attributes as part of admission screening in NA programs.

The results of research evaluating utility of admission criteria factors leads to a growing body of evidence related to establishing research-based admission selection criteria for NA programs, which provide significant predictive value of positive student progression to graduation. Results also help inform decisions made by anesthesia program faculty and administrators about how to best weight admission criteria if a weighting system is used. A priority program evaluation strategy should include evaluation of the relationship between GRE scores and years of critical care experience as well as academic progression of students enrolled in their own programs.

DOCTORAL PROGRAMS IN NURSING

Doctor of Nursing Practice and Doctor of Philosophy/Nursing Science

In its landmark report, *The Future of Nursing: Leading Change, Advancing Health,* the IOM (2010) called for doubling the number of doctoral prepared nurses by 2020 in an effort to alleviate the shortage of nurses prepared to address the nation's current and future health care needs. Schools were urged to increase diversity and to design academic programs in which nurses could obtain advanced degrees in a "seamless" manner.

In addition, the IOM encouraged the nursing profession to reexamine its traditional research-focused doctoral programs, such as those leading to the PhD and doctor of nursing science (DNS). Increased attention also was paid to DNP programs. Both practice- and research-focused doctoral programs are essential for meeting the nation's health care needs. Because these two doctoral programs prepare graduates for different, yet complementary, roles, they require diverse program elements, resources, and evaluation. The AACN (2014) has outlined these differences based on program objectives, programs of study, student career interests, faculty, resources, and program outcomes.

Practice-Focused Doctorate in Nursing: DNP

As a practice-focused doctorate, the DNP prepares advanced practice nurses to "improve patient outcomes and translate research into practice" (AACN, 2014, p. 1). The DNP was proposed as the terminal degree for advanced practice nurses including NPs, clinical nurse specialists, certified nurse-midwives, certified registered nurse anesthetists, and others with interest to "implement the science developed by nurse researchers" (AACN, 2015c, p. 1). In 2015, the AACN's white paper, *Current Issues and Clarifying Recommendations* (AACN, 2015e), clarified elements essential for practice-focused doctoral programs in nursing. Program components such as the curriculum, final DNP scholarly project, clinical practice hours, and program length were clarified, as much variation was noted among DNP programs. Having consistency among these key elements is essential in program evaluation.

As of March 2015, there were 264 DNP programs in 48 states and the District of Columbia; 60 programs were in progress (AACN, 2015c). Since 2006, the number of DNP programs have nearly tripled (AACN, 2015c). Both student enrollments and graduations have increased about 25% from 2013 to 2014 (AACN, 2015c).

Research-Focused Doctorates: PhD and DNS

The PhD/DNS degrees are research-focused doctorates that "prepare nurses at the highest level of nursing science to conduct research to advance the science of nursing" (AACN, 2014, p. 1). The PhD in nursing has existed since the 1950s (Broome, Halstead, Pesut, Rawl, & Boland, 2011) with quality indicators published in the 1980s (Jamann, 1985) and updated in 2010 (AACN, 2010). As of March 2015, 134 PhD programs were active in the United States (AACN, 2015c). Since 2006, the growth in new PhD programs has been much slower than that reported for DNP programs; 31 programs began from 2006 to 2014 (AACN, 2015c). Doctoral enrollment in research-focused programs from 2010 to 2014 increased by nearly 15% (N = 688) while graduations grew about 39% (N = 210) over that period (Fang, Li, Arietti, & Trautman, 2015).

Evolving changes in doctoral education demands ongoing assessment and systematic evaluation. Particular attention should be paid to: (1) faculty numbers and qualifications, (2) curriculum and role-specific competencies, and (3) program outcomes.

Faculty Numbers and Qualifications

Doctoral programs must have a sufficient number of faculty who are qualified to meet the needs of the nursing program (CCNE, 2013). In fact, the nurse faculty shortage has caused schools of nursing to limit their student enrollments (AACN, 2015d). In 2014, nursing programs cited faculty shortages among the primary reason for not offering admission to 1,844 qualified applicants (AACN, 2015d).

Although multiple strategies are currently in place to address the faculty shortage (AACN, 2015d), several researchers have raised capacity issues in schools given the rapid growth in DNP programs. In a national survey of 554 nursing faculty teaching in U.S. PhD and DNP programs, Smeltzer et al. (2015) noted that faculty who taught in DNP programs differed significantly on several characteristics from their colleagues who taught in either PhD or combined DNP/PhD programs. The faculty teaching in DNP programs had fewer years as educators, were employed fewer years in their current positions, and spent less time weekly on scholarship. DNP faculty spent more time teaching each week compared to their research-focused colleagues. Given the rapid growth in DNP programs, the authors expressed concern for the future of scholarship and science for the nursing profession. Similarly, Minnick, Norman, and Donaghey (2013) also questioned DNP program capacity issues based on the results of their survey of 130 DNP programs. Their findings reflected a wide range of variation in how schools had implemented their DNP programs and the role-specific requirements.

Since faculty qualifications differ for teaching in the two types of doctoral programs, attention needs to be paid to faculty development. According to the AACN, faculty teaching in DNP programs should possess the following qualifications: a practice or research doctorate in nursing, expertise in teaching, leadership experience in the role and practice area, and expertise in practice congruent with the focus of the academic program (AACN, 2014, p. 1). Conversely, faculty teaching in PhD/DNS programs should hold a research doctorate in nursing or related fields, leadership experience in an area of sustained research focus, and a high level of expertise in research that is consistent with the focus of the academic program (AACN, 2014, p. 1). The current and future faculty shortage poses an additional challenge to meeting current and future needs for appropriately qualified doctoral nursing faculty.

Curriculum Content and Competencies

Since DNP and PhD/DNS programs prepare nurse leaders for two complementary, yet different, roles, faculty must design role-specific curricula and obtain resources—such as clinical sites and preceptors—that will enable graduates to develop their expected roles. Curriculum standards for the DNP degree are outlined in *The Essentials of Doctoral Education for Advanced Nursing Practice* (AACN, 2006), which focuses attention on practice-based competencies such as evidence-based practice, interprofessional collaboration, population health, and organizational/systems leadership. A DNP project is required as a program-end deliverable that provides evidence of the student's ability to synthesize curriculum essentials; this project can assume various practice-based forms, among them clinical practice changes, program evaluations, and quality improvement initiatives (AACN, 2006).

DNP curricula have traditionally been shorter than PhD programs, with a recommended post-MSN DNP full-time program at a minimum of 12 months (AACN, 2006; 2015e). Various models have been proposed to facilitate timely progression to the DNP, among them beginning with a master's degree as a clinical nurse leader and taking additional specialization courses in order to advance to the DNP, as well as beginning with a BSN to the DNP (Chism, 2010).

Quality standards for research-focused doctoral programs have existed since the 1980s (Jamann, 1985) with quality indicators published by the AACN (2010) in *The Research-Focused Doctoral Program in Nursing: Pathways to Excellence*, which details the role, expected outcomes, and core curricular elements. Curricula should focus on enabling students to develop competencies to advance nursing science. Content in PhD programs typically includes areas such as history and philosophy of science, research methods, and scholarship-focused opportunities such as grant development and publications. The program-end synthesis product for PhD students is original research in the form of a dissertation (AACN, 2010). The AACN (2010) offers eight pathways that enable timely transition to a PhD.

Recent attention has been paid to maintaining the quality of PhD curricula content with a focus on the inclusion of emerging areas of science (Breslin, Sebastain, Trautman, & Rosseter, 2015). Wyman and Henly (2015) reviewed the curriculum content posted on the websites of 120 PhD/DNS programs in the United States to determine the extent to which AACN quality indicators and emerging areas of science were evident (AACN, 2010). Results revealed that many PhD programs included outdated guidelines. While some core elements existed, most of the AACN requirements were inconsistently represented. Little attention was paid to content aligned with current science such as genetics and nursing science priorities such as symptom management.

Program Outcomes

DNP programs are accredited by either the CCNE (2013) or the Accreditation Commission for Education in Nursing (ACEN, 2013). PhD/DNS programs do not have a similar accreditation body, but rather, follow their institutional policies regarding external review (AACN, 2014). Administrators of doctoral programs need to conduct ongoing and systematic evaluation of their programs based on each doctoral-specific role. Program outcomes for the DNP should focus on "healthcare improvements and contributions via practice, policy change, and practice scholarship" (AACN, 2014, p. 1). Conversely, research-focused doctoral programs should track the "development of new knowledge and scholarly products that provide the foundation for the advancement of nursing science" (AACN, 2014, p. 1).

Evidence should be collected from various stakeholders and sources, and incorporated as part of ongoing quality improvement. Alumni and employers can offer insight into the role-specific productivity of graduates (AACN, 2015c). Broome et al. (2011) tracked benchmarks such as successful course completion, pass rates on qualifying exams, and final dissertation defenses when evaluating their PhD program. The DNP project is a similar benchmark.

Broome et al. (2011) described a process and outcome evaluation that they conducted for their PhD program. Although their program was a distance-accessible one, their approach included clear program outcomes and competencies aligned with national quality indicators. This example illustrates a comprehensive model that can be used for both DNP and PhD program evaluation. Through alumni feedback, the authors also focused on identifying best practices for mentoring PhD students to develop their researcher role.

SUMMARY

This chapter has presented the latest evidence-based research on aspects of program assessment and evaluation pertinent to RN to BSN, accelerated second career programs, nurse practitioner, nurse anesthesia, and doctoral programs in nursing. Program administrators and faculty charged with program evaluation responsibilities can incorporate this information into the design of assessment and evaluation processes in support of continual program and performance improvement initiatives.

References

Accreditation Commission for Education in Nursing (ACEN). (2013). *ACEN accreditation manual*. Retrieved from http://www.acenursing.org/accreditation-manual/

American Association of Colleges of Nursing. (2006). *The essentials of doctoral education for advanced nursing practice*. Retrieved from www.aacn.nche.edu/publications/position/DNPEssentials.pdf

American Association of Colleges of Nursing. (2010). *The research-focused doctoral program in nursing: Pathways to excellence*. Retrieved from www.aacn.nche.edu/education-resources/PhDTaskForceReport.pdf

American Association of Colleges of Nursing. (2012). *White paper: Expectations for practice experiences in the RN to baccalaureate curriculum*. Retrieved from www.aacn.nche.

edu/aacn-publications/white-papers/RN-BSN-White-Paper.pdf

American Association of Colleges of Nursing. (2014). *Key differences between DNP and PhD/DNS Programs.* Retrieved from www.aacn.nche.edu/dnp/ContrastGrid.pdf

American Association of Colleges of Nursing. (2015a). *Fact sheet: Accelerated baccalaureate and master's degrees in nursing.* Retrieved from http://www.aacn.nche.edu/students/accelerated-nursing-programs

American Association of Colleges of Nursing. (2015b). *Fact sheet: Degree completion programs for Registered Nurses: RN to Master's degree and RN to Baccalaureate degree.* Retrieved from www.aacn.nche.edu/media-relations/fact-sheets/degree-completion-Programs

American Association of Colleges of Nursing. (2015c). *Fact sheet: The doctor of nursing practice (DNP).* Retrieved from http://www.aacn.nche.edu/media-relations/fact-sheets/dnp

American Association of Colleges of Nursing. (2015d). *Nursing faculty shortage fact sheet.* Retrieved from http://www.aacn.nche.edu/media-relations/fact-sheets/nursing-faculty-shortage

American Association of Colleges of Nursing. (2015e). *New white paper on the DNP: Current issues and clarifying recommendations.* Retrieved from http://www.aacn.nche.edu/news/articles/2015/dnp-white-paper

American Association of Colleges of Nursing. (2015f). *White paper: Current state of APRN clinical education.* Retrieved from www.aacn.nche.edu/APRN-White-Paper.pdf

American Association of Nurse Anesthetists. (2015). *Timeline of AANA History, Pre-AANA.* Retrieved from www.aana.com/resources2/archives-library/Pages/Timeline-of-AANA-History-Pre-AANA.aspx

American Association of Nurse Practitioners. (2015). *NP Fact Sheet.* Retrieved from www.aanp.org/all-about-nps/np-fact-sheet

APRN Consensus Work Group and National Council of State Boards of Nursing APRN Advisory Committee. (2008). *Consensus model for APRN regulation: Licensure, accreditation, certification & education.* Retrieved from http://www.aacn.nche.edu/education-resources/APRNReport.pdf

Boellaard, M. R., Brandt, C. L., & Zorn, C. R. (2015). Faculty to faculty: Advice for educators teaching in accelerated second baccalaureate degree nursing programs. *Journal of Nursing Education, 54,* 343–346. doi:10.3928/01484834-20150515-06

Brandt, C. L., Boellaard, M. R., & Zorn, C. R. (2013). Experiences and emotions of faculty teaching in accelerated second baccalaureate degree nursing programs. *Journal of Nursing Education, 52,* 377–382. doi:10.3982/01484834-20130613-02

Brandt, C. L., Boellaard, M. R., & Zorn, C. R. (2015). The faculty voice: Teaching in accelerated second baccalaureate degree nursing programs. *Journal of Nursing Education, 54,* 241–247. doi: 10.3928/0148484834-20150417-01

Breslin, E., Sebastain, J., Trautman, D., & Rosseter, R. (2015). Sustaining excellence and relevance in PhD nursing education. *Nursing Outlook, 63,* 428–531. doi:10.1016/j.outlook.2015.04.002

Broome, M. E., Halstead, J. A., Pesut, D. J., Rawl, S. M., & Boland, D.L. (2011). Evaluating the outcomes of a distance-accessible PhD program. *Journal of Professional Nursing, 27,* 69–77. doi:10.1016/j.profnurs.2010.09.011

Bureau of Labor Statistics (2014). *Occupational Outlook Handbook: Nurse Anesthetists, Nurse Midwives, and Nurse Practitioner.* Retrieved from www.bls.gov/ooh/health-care/nurse-anesthetists-nurse-midwives-and-nurse-practitioners.htm

Burns, S. M. (2011). Predicting academic progression for student registered nurse anesthetists. *AANA Journal, 79,* 193–201.

Cangelosi, P. R. (2013). Teaching experiences of second degree accelerated baccalaureate nursing faculty. *International Journal of Nursing Education Scholarship, 10,* 275–281. doi 10.1515/ijnes-2013-0043

Chism, L. A. (2010). Overview of the doctor of nursing practice degree. In L. A. Chism (Ed.) *The doctor of nursing practice: A guidebook for role development and professional issues* (pp. 3–31). Sudbury, MA: Jones and Barlett.

Collins, S., & Callahan, M. F. (2014). A call for change: Clinical evaluation of student registered nurse anesthetists. *AANA Journal, 82*(1), 65–72.

Commission on Collegiate Nursing Education. (2013). *Standards for accreditation of baccalaureate and graduate nursing programs.* Retrieved from http://www.aacn.nche.edu/ccne-accreditation/standards-procedures-resources/baccalaureate-graduate/standards

Council on Accreditation of Nurse Anesthesia Educational Programs. (2015). *Accreditation.* Retrieved from http://home.coa.us.com/accreditation/Pages/default.aspx

Driessnack, M., Mobily, P., Stineman, A., Montgomery, L. A., Clow, T., & Elsbach, S. (2011). We are different: Learning needs of accelerated second degree nursing students. *Nurse Educator, 36,* 214–218. doi: 10.1097/NNE.obo13e3182297c90

Fang, D., Bednash, G. P., & DeWitty, V. P. (2012). The growth of accelerated BSN and MSN programs in the United States: A national perspective (pp. 227–242). In Zhan, L., & Finch, L. P. (2012). *Accelerated education in nursing: Challenges, strategies, and future directions.* New York, NY: Springer.

Fang, D., Li, Y., Arietti, R., & Trautman, D. E. (2015). *2014–2015 Enrollment and graduations in baccalaureate and graduate programs in nursing.* Washington, DC: American Association of Colleges of Nursing.

Frost, J. (2015). *Assessing outcome performance competencies in physical therapy: Future directions of credentialing research in nursing.* Retrieved from http://www.iom.edu/~/media/Files/Activity%%20Files/Workforce/FutureDirectionsCNRworkshop/NCR%20Workshop%20Presentations/2%20Frost%20COPYRIGHT%20APPROVED.pdf

Hooper, J. I., McEwen, M., & Mancini, M. (2013). A regulatory challenge: Creating a metric for quality RN-to-BSN programs. *Journal of Nursing Regulation, 4*(2), 34–38. doi: 10.1016/S2155-8256(15)30156-3

Institute of Medicine (IOM). (2010). *The future of nursing: Leading change, advancing health.* Retrieved from http://www.iom.edu/Reports/2010/The-Future-of-Nursing-Leading-Change-Advancing-Health.aspx

Jamann, J. S. (1985). Proceedings of doctoral programs in nursing: Consensus for quality. *Journal of Professional Nursing, 1,* 90–121.

Kemsley, M., McCausland, L., Feigenbaum, J., & Riegle, E. (2011). Analysis of graduates' perceptions of an accelerated bachelor of science program in nursing. *Journal of Professional Nursing, 27,* 50–58. doi: 10.1016/j.profnurs.2010.09.006

Mancini, M., Ashwill, J., & Cipher, D. J. (2015). A comparative analysis of demographic and academic success characteristics of online and on-campus RN-to-BSN students. *Journal of Professional Nursing, 31,* 71–76. doi:10.1016/j.profnurs.2014.05.008

Matthews, M. B., & Travis, L. L. (1994). Research on the baccalaureate completion process for RNs. *Annual Review of Nursing Research, 12,* 149–171. doi:10.1177/07417130122087313

McEwen, M., White, M. J., Pullis, B. R., & Krawtz, S. (2014). Essential content in RN-BSN programs. *Journal of Professional Nursing, 30,* 333–340. doi: 10.1016/j.profnurs.2013.10.003

Minnick, A. F., Norman, L. D., & Donaghey, B. (2013). Defining and describing capacity issues in U.S. doctor of nursing practice programs. *Nursing Outlook, 61,* 93–101. http://dx.doi.org/10.1016/j.outlook.2012.07.011

National Task Force on Quality Nurse Practitioner Education (2012). *Criteria for evaluation of nurse practitioner programs* (4th ed.). Washington, DC: National Organization of Nurse Practitioner Faculties. Retrieved from http://www.aacn.nche.edu/education-resources/evalcriteria2012.pdf

Newton, S. E., & Moore, G. (2013). Critical thinking skills of basic baccalaureate and accelerated second-degree nursing students. *Nursing Education Perspectives, 14,* 154–158.

Nugent, E., & LaRocco, S. (2014). Comprehensive review of an accelerated program. *Dimensions of Critical Care Nursing, 33,* 226–233. doi: 10.1097/DCC.0000000000000054

O'Brien, B., & Renner, A. (2000). Nurses online: Career mobility for registered nurses. *Journal of Professional Nursing, 16,* 13–20. doi: 10.1016/S8755-7223(00)80007-1

Oermann, M. H., Poole-Dawkins, K., Alvarez, M. T., Foster, B. B., & O'Sullivan, R. (2010). Manager's perspectives of new graduates of accelerated nursing programs: How do they compare with other graduates? *Journal of Continuing Education in Nursing, 41*, 394–400. doi: 10.3928/00220124-20100601-01

Oermann, M. H., Alvarez, M. T., O'Sullivan, R., & Foster, B. B. (2010). Performance satisfaction, and transition into practice of graduates of accelerated nursing programs. *Journal for Nurses in Staff Development, 26*, 192–199. doi: 10.1097/NND.0b013e31819b5c3a.

Ortega, K. H., Burns, S. M., Hussey, L. C., Schmidt, J., & Austin, P. N. (2013). Predicting success in nurse anesthesia programs: An evidence-based review of admission criteria. *AANA Journal, 81*, 183–189.

Payne, L. K., Glaspie, T., & Rosser, C. (2014). Comparison of select outcomes between traditional and accelerated BSN programs: A Pilot study. *Nursing Education Perspectives, 35*, 332–334.

Penprase, B. (2012). Perceptions, orientation, and transition into nursing practice of accelerated second-degree nursing program graduates. *Journal of Continuing Education in Nursing, 43*, 29–36. doi: 10.3928/00220124-20110315-02

Penprase, B., & Harris, M. A. (2013). Accelerated second-degree nursing students: Predictors of graduation and NCLEX-RN first time pass rates. *Nurse Educator, 38*, 26–29. doi: 10.1097/NNE.0b013e318276df16

Penprase, B., Mileto, L., Bittinger, A., Hranchook, A. M., Atchley, J. A., Bergakker, S.A., ... Franson, H.E. (2012). The use of high-fidelity simulation in the admission process: One nurse anesthesia program's experience. *AANA Journal, 80*(1), 43–48.

Rafferty, M., & Lindell, D. (2011). How nurse managers rate the clinical competencies of accelerated (second-degree) nursing graduates. *Journal of Nursing Education, 50*, 355–358. doi: 10.3928/01484834-20110228-07

Raines, D. A. (2010). Nursing practice competency of accelerated bachelor of science in nursing program students. *Journal of Profes-sional Nursing, 26*, 162–167. doi: 10.1016/j.profnurs.2009.12.004

Roach, K. E., Frost, J.S., Francis, N. J., Giles, S., & Nordrum, A. D. (2012). Validation of the revised physical therapist clinical perfor-mance instrument (PT CPI): Version 2006. *Physical Therapy, 92*, 416–428.

Robert, T. E., Pomarico, C. A., & Nolan, M. (2011). Assessing faculty integration of adult learning needs in second-degree nursing education. *Nursing Education Perspectives, 32*(4), 14–17.

Robertson, S., Canary, C.W., Orr, M., Herberg, P., & Rutledge, D. N. (2010). Factors related to progression and graduation rates for RN-to-Bachelor of Science in nursing programs: Searching for realistic benchmarks. *Journal of Professional Nursing, 26*, 99–107. doi: 10.1016/j.profnurs.2009.09.003

Smeltzer, S. C., Sharts-Hopko, N. C., Cantrell, M. A., Heverly, M. A., Nthenge, S., & Jenkinson, A. (2015). A profile of U.S. nurs-ing faculty in research- and practice-focused doctoral education. *Journal of Nursing Schol-arship, 47*, 178–185. doi: 10.1111/jnu.12123

Stokowski, L. A. (2011). Overhauling nurs-ing education. *Medscape Nurses News.* Retrieved from http://www.medscape.com/viewarticle/736236

Stuenkel, D., Nelson, D., Malloy, S. & Cohen, J. (2011). Challenges, changes, and collabo-ration: Evaluation of an accelerated BSN program. *Nurse Educator, 36*(2), 70–75. doi:10.1097/NNEOb013e31820c7cf7

Texas Board of Nursing (2011). Differentiated essential competencies of graduates of Texas nursing programs. Retrieved from www.bon.texas.gov/pdfs/publication_pdfs/delc-2010.pdf

Wros, P., Wheeler, P., & Jones, M. (2011). *Cur-riculum planning for baccalaureate nursing programs.* In Keating, S. B. (Ed.): *Curriculum development and evaluation in nursing.* (2nd ed., pp. 209–240). New York, NY: Springer.

Wyman. J. F., & Henly, S. J. (2015). PhD pro-grams in nursing in the United States: Vis-ibility of American Association of Colleges of Nursing core curricular elements and emerging areas of science. *Nursing Outlook, 63*, 390–397. http://dx.doi.org/10.1016/j.outlook.2014.11.003

11

Managing Organizational Change Effectively

Sharon Kumm, MN, MS, CNE
Nelda Godfrey, PhD, ACNS-BC, FAAN

Change is a reality in all organizations, with many organizations having continual change. Some organizations are more successful in transitioning and successfully managing change, while others either are unable to enact change or fail to sustain it. In this chapter, we discuss change and leadership theories that are particularly useful in academic environments, the change process itself and factors that can impede or foster change, a systems approach to evaluation, making organizational decisions based on assessment and evaluation data, considerations in identifying and maximizing stakeholder investment in the change process, and strategies for balancing resources and costs when implementing organizational change.

THEORIES OF CHANGE

Initially, change models and theories focused on the process of change. However, with a greater understanding of the process and the effects of change, new theories have emerged that address both process issues and the psychological stress that individuals encounter. Two theories are particularly useful in understanding and guiding change in contemporary academic settings: the Bridges Transition Model of Change and Complexity Leadership Theory.

Bridges Transition Model of Change

Bridges (2009) defines change as the process that occurs whether the individual agrees or not and transition as the psychological processes that occur as the individual experiences and internalizes change. The Bridges transition model occurs in three stages: letting go, the neutral zone, and new beginnings. In the letting-go phase, the individual recognizes and grieves over what will be lost—security, knowledge of one's place in the organization—and faces uncertainty. New procedures must be learned. The neutral zone is a period in which the traditional methods are gone, and the new structure is not fully in place. This is a critical period of realignment and repatterning, with individuals experiencing high levels of anxiety. In the new-beginnings phase, individuals have a new sense of purpose, with excitement and high energy to make the new processes work. In each phase, individuals need encouragement and support. Bridges posits that, for change to be successful, letting go of the old and acknowledging the loss are both essential. Change may happen quickly, but dealing with the psychological aspect takes longer (Bridges, 2009).

Complexity Leadership Theory

Complexity leadership theory recognizes the organizational dynamics and continual change of today's work environments (Uhl-Bien & Marion, 2011). This theory suggests that change occurs through both formal and informal processes and requires complex interactions. With this theory, change results from "local actions that occur simultaneously around the system linking up with one another to produce powerful emergent phenomena" (Uhl-Bien & Marion, p. 469). Emergence is the process by which interactions in systems (or subsystems) lead to change or the development of new ideas (Wood & Butt, 2014).

For change to occur, administrators need to share information and catalyze lower-level workers to generate emergence and adaptation. Complex adaptive leaders are expected to function at the intersection of administration and adaptation, where the administrative function focuses on efficiency and control and the adaptive role on innovation. Adaptive leadership encourages empowerment, trust, psychological safety, networking, collaboration, and creativity, which promote moving innovative outcomes into the formal system. This empowerment allows for bottom-up change (Uhl-Bien & Marion, 2011) in spite of increasing levels of complexity in the environment. Leaders focus on creating environments and conditions that are conducive to emergence.

FACTORS THAT INFLUENCE CHANGE

Given the impact of systems theory thinking and a life sciences orientation on nursing practice and education, we define the change process as *the impact on the patterns, structures, and processes that occur within an open system* (Capra, 1996) *and that interact externally with other types of systems* (Burke, 2014). These systems can be interdisciplinary in nature and can have wide or limited impact. Therefore, the change that occurs in organizations embracing a systematic approach to assessment and evaluation will likely yield patterns and movement that reflect the complexity and nonlinearity of larger, open systems.

Readiness for Change

One could infer that the best results for instituting change will come from accurate assessment and appropriate incorporation of assessment data in planning and implementation. Yet, organizations and individuals struggle with how to reliably and accurately measure readiness for change. Part of the reason that this is difficult is that change exists at two levels—individual and organizational—and these two levels are linked. Readiness occurs both structurally (circumstances and materials required) and psychologically (capacity to process and accept change; Burke, 2014). Holt, Helfrich, Hall, and Weiner (2010) define four key constructs that constitute readiness:

1. Individual psychological factors that reflect the extent to which individuals hold key beliefs regarding the proposed change, recognize a problem needs to be addressed, and agree with the changes required

2. Individual structural factors including individuals' knowledge, skills, and ability to perform once the change is implemented

3. Organizational psychological factors regarding how effectively members work together toward a common goal

4. Organizational structural factors related to human (champions and leaders) and material resources (information technology, equipment, and finances), communication channels, and formal policy

Readiness to Change Assessment Tools

A number of tools are available to assess readiness for change. The Organizational Change Management Readiness Guide (Information Technology Leadership Academy, 2014) is one example that is easy to use, comprehensive, and accessible online. Originally developed to assist informational technologists in California to prepare for a change in fiscal management, it is generalizable to most organizational changes because the aim is to prepare organizations to integrate and align people, processes, culture, and strategies. This tool is comprised of five pillars: communication, readiness, sponsorship, stakeholder management, and training. Each pillar has five subcomponents that can be scored on a Likert scale of 1 (strongly disagree) to 6 (strongly agree). An average score below four in any category means that the organization is not fully prepared for change, and leaders must communicate the need for change more effectively and find champions for the change (Information Technology Leadership Academy, 2014).

Change Resistance

Change is a complex process embedded in social interactions and emotions. The emotional component of change is related to both change resistance and fatigue. Change resistance, intentional actions that sabotage organizational change, has been associated with failure of change efforts and may be triggered by a repeated history of change failures. These behaviors may be verbal (cynical remarks, critical questioning, and denying need) or nonverbal (eye rolling or smirks) aimed directly at the change leader or in informal conversations. Resistance has the benefit of stimulating discussion about the need for the change (McMillan & Perron, 2013).

Change Fatigue

Unlike the blatant behavior of resistance, change fatigue is passive, with behaviors of disengagement, apathy, and ambivalence, and often goes unrecognized. Fatigue is associated with rapid and continuous changes and can result in failure to sustain the change. Methods to recognize or decrease change fatigue and resistance are similar. Assessment

---

BOX 11.1

Strategies to Positively Influence Change in Schools of Nursing

Developing a unity of purpose

Co-creating mission and vision statements

Seeking outside consultation/guidance

Expressing a unifying leadership culture by formal unit leader (dean/director or team leader)

Gathering and communicating the data in ways that faculty can understand

Tying change to external influences: accreditation standards, funding formulas, boards of nursing, state educational governing boards

Using a timeline and taking "small steps" in accomplishing the whole task

Identifying a faculty leader to help guide the change by convening meetings, setting agendas

Using small group works with outputs reported to the larger group

---

of readiness to change will identify if front-line workers, for example, nursing faculty, are prepared and think that the necessary processes are in place. Participatory management can foster accountability and ownership of change initiatives (McMillan & Perron, 2013).

Strategies to Positively Influence Change

More specifically, targeted strategies may be needed to facilitate the desired change. Box 11.1 presents strategies that have been effective in academic nursing settings. The effort needed to make and support changes in an organization is not to be underestimated; in many cases, organizational change requires a culture shift that may require each individual to think about and perhaps redefine values such as shared purpose, self-interest, respect, and tradition (Lee & Cosgrove, 2014).

Lencioni (2012) discusses the singular advantage of *organizational health* in successful businesses, underscoring the need to first build a cohesive leadership team and next to create clarity, overcommunicate clarity, and reinforce clarity. The leadership team needs to communicate messages clearly and strategically with those in the organization. Table 11.1 presents methods for engaging stakeholders in change. Communication is inherently or directly present within each strategy to engage stakeholders.

A SYSTEMS APPROACH TO EVALUATION

Systems theory proposes that there are universal principles of organizations that are true for all systems: The whole is greater than the sum of its parts; the parts are interrelated; and parts cannot be understood in isolation from the whole. Systems are goal oriented and have inputs, outputs, and feedback about the outputs, and must respond to changes in the environment in which they are situated (Chand, 2015). A systems approach to

TABLE 11.1

Methods to Engage Stakeholders

	Inform	Consult	Involve	Collaborate	Empower
Bulletins/Formal memos/Letters	X				
Displays/Exhibits	X	X			
Email/Fax/Phone	X	X		X	X
Focus Groups		X	X		
Forums		X	X	X	
Information Hotline	X				
Interviews		X	X		
Meetings	X	X	X	X	X
Negotiations		X		X	
Newsletters/Postcards/Fact sheets	X				
Open House	X	X	X	X	
Questionnaire/Survey		X			
Walking tours/Site visits		X	X		
Website	X	X		X	
Workshop		X	X	X	X

Adapted from Yang, J., Shen, P. Q., Bourne, L., Mo, C. M. F., & Xue, X. (2011). A typology of operational approaches for stakeholder analysis and engagement: Findings from Hong Kong and Australia. *Construction Management and Economics, 29,* 145–162.

evaluation requires looking at the whole and the parts. The subsystems need to be studied in their interrelationships rather than in isolation. The systems approach to evaluation examines the organizational structure, information exchange, planning and control mechanisms, and roles and functions of faculty, administrators, staff and others in the school, as well as the subsystems (departments).

The ultimate purpose of evaluation is to make data-driven decisions that lead to improved outcomes or performance. All components of the evaluation need to be aligned with the objectives and expectations that the organization values and decisions that need to be made as a result of the findings. Systematic evaluation identifies what went right or wrong, as well as why and how to modify those factors so that it can meet the intended objectives (Guerra-Lopez, 2012). Evaluation can provide a systematic framework that aligns stakeholders, evaluation purposes, desired outcomes, and all activities so that the evaluation product provides a clear direction for improvement. Since all variables in organizations are interdependent, systems-based evaluation processes are needed to determine the ultimate outcomes and value-added results.

The Impact Monitoring and Evaluation Process developed by Guerra-Lopez (2012) is a method of systems evaluation. It includes these stages:

- *Identify stakeholders.* Stakeholders include groups who finance the effort, those carrying out the functions, and those who are impacted by the evaluation. Each group should be represented on the evaluation team, and the expectations of each group should be determined at the beginning. Guerra-Lopez (2012) indicates that "if you do not align your efforts with stakeholder expectations from the start, it is very unlikely you ever meet those expectations" (p. 83).

- *Determine key decisions and objectives.* The decisions that should be made are relevant to the broader performance management system and are linked to organizational objectives. The relative worth of any intervention or solution should be contingent on whether it is helping or hindering achievement of the organizational objectives and desired impact. Once the decisions and objectives are clarified, the overarching questions that will guide the evaluation will become clear.

- *Derive measurable indicators.* Sound decisions are based on relevant, reliable, valid, and complete data. Data should be collected on key performance indicators (e.g., employment of graduates and student satisfaction). The questions derived in the previous stage determine which key indicators to select.

- *Identify appropriate data sources.* The data sought determine the source. Excellent resources include past studies done in the organization, strategic and operational plans, annual reports, project plans, consulting studies, and performance reports. Conflicting data from various sources or missing data are important to identify so that methods can be developed to collect this information in the future.

- *Select data collection instruments.* Evaluation efforts should use the right tools for the types of data to be collected. Both qualitative and quantitative data may be required. Tools used in quality improvement are useful to organize and analyze data, for example, process mapping, resource allocation, Pareto charting, root-cause analysis, generating alternative solutions, double-loop learning, prioritizing solutions, and creating action plans. The use of these tools depends on the phase of the change process (Table 11.2).

- *Select data analysis approaches.* Analysis of data includes discovering patterns, developing arguments to support conclusions, deciding how to improve performance, and recognizing the impact that evaluation efforts have on students, faculty, staff, and other stakeholders.

- *Continuous feedback and action.* Communication about evaluation data, interpretations of the data, patterns, trends, alternative courses of action, and relationship to the objectives is essential. Effective communication promotes engagement and decreases resistance (Guerra-Lopez, 2012).

TABLE 11.2

Techniques and Tools Useful in Each Stage of Change Process

Change Process	Tools or Techniques
Assess the need for change	Brainstorming, Pareto charts (ranked bar chart that indicates frequency), process mapping (visualize the inputs, process, and outputs involved in delivering a product related to the initiative)
Collect and analyze data	Check sheets, control and run charts (visualize how data change over time), force field analysis (identify forces that may affect the new initiative), cause-and-effect diagrams (fish bones)
Explore alternatives and select solution	Check sheets, control or run charts, force field analysis, histograms, cause-and-effect diagrams, scatter diagrams
Implement change	Process mapping, logic model (graphic model of the causal relationships among resources, activities, outputs and outcomes of a program or initiative)
Evaluate change	Control and run charts, scatter diagrams, histograms, check sheets, Pareto charts

It is essential to keep in mind that the purpose of evaluation is to improve decision-making to support actions that result in measurable performance improvement and value-added impact on the nursing program, school, and society. Stakeholder support is essential because stakeholders may hold the authority for the evaluation, provide access to resources, and identify criteria for success. Goals, objectives, and performance indicators and targets must be considered in the context of strategic and operational outcomes desired by the institution.

MAKING ORGANIZATIONAL DECISIONS BASED ON ASSESSMENT AND EVALUATION DATA

Learning organizations perform best when decisions are made in a collaborative setting and supported by knowledge derived from operating data. Educators are not only being confronted with more data but also with different kinds of data from multiple sources. Data should no longer be only for accountability, but to stimulate and inform continuous improvement (Mandinach, 2012). Data are meaningless until they are put in context. Data may be used for instructional or administrative decision-making and should be part of an ongoing cycle of improvement. Supports and resources are needed to establish and sustain a data culture within schools of nursing. Barriers to data use include lack of release time for analysis and planning, and lack of knowledge of analysis.

Data Driven Decision-Making (DDDM) is founded on the continuum of data to knowledge. Six skills are involved in this continuum. At the data level, users collect and organize data. At the information level, users analyze and summarize information, and at the knowledge level, users synthesize and prioritize knowledge. Following this, users decide on an action, implement the action, and evaluate the impact. This process is similar to the nursing process and the Plan-Do-Study-Act cycle of quality improvement. Mandinach (2012) identified the key components of DDDM to be technology and data literacy. As the amount of data available increases, educators need to know how to collect data using technology and use data literacy to manage and analyze the data to develop solutions.

Since DDDM comes from quality management and management science, it uses many of the same tools to collect and analyze organizational data (e.g., financial, student enrollment statistics) and other data (assessments, core measures) to inform decisions. Each institution will decide on the data that are useful in decision-making in their school, such as performance measures and benchmarks. DDDM is a systematic process to generate useful and relevant knowledge by combining data and situational context (e.g., culture of the organization, institutional past practices, reliability and accuracy of the data, stakeholder requirements). DDDM generates the key performance indicators to enable administrators and faculty to prioritize strategies, allocate resources, govern the pace of implementation, and provide feedback and monitoring to benchmark performance against independent standards of excellence (Callery, 2012).

The complexity of aligning organizational structures, resources, and programs with new directives often requires a new skill set for administration, faculty, and staff. To sustain change, champions are essential—these are people who believe that the change will benefit the organization and its mission. Champions can be administrators, faculty, or staff as informal champions or assigned as task force leaders (Callery, 2012).

IDENTIFYING AND MAXIMIZING STAKEHOLDER INVESTMENT

While stakeholders are identified as important components of systems evaluation, specialized attention will be needed with the stakeholders to effectively lead organizational change. Stakeholders are individuals or agencies, both internal and external, that are affected by or affect your organization's products or activities. The major internal stakeholders in education changes include faculty, students, and staff. Administration may be considered an internal or external stakeholder. Stakeholder management has several key steps:

- Identify relevant stakeholders.
- Determine the level of influence and interest for each stakeholder. Ask if the stakeholder will be a champion for or feel threatened by the proposed change.
- Engage the stakeholders as early as possible. Reach out to key stakeholders at the inception of the evaluation, and communicate frequently to build trust and create enthusiasm.
- Communicate frequently using a variety of methods. The method of communication depends on the influence and interest of the stakeholder and the purpose of the communication. Stakeholders with a high level of

interest and influence may need to have face-to-face meetings interspersed with written communication. Stakeholders with less interest may be kept informed with mailings and electronic means, such as websites. Additional methods of communication are included in Table 11.2.

- Solicit feedback from key stakeholders about major decisions. The frequency of obtaining feedback depends on the interest and influence of the stakeholder. It is also important to communicate to the stakeholders how their input has been used in the school.

USING EVALUATION DATA TO BETTER UNDERSTAND ORGANIZATIONAL RESOURCES AND COSTS

The case for gathering quality assessment and evaluation data along with the institutional benefit of a robust review of the data analysis has been addressed in preceding chapters. In this section, we explain the relationships among resources, costs, and data and how the findings from the analysis phase of program evaluation can substantially add to the understanding of nursing units' leaders and faculty members as they successfully implement key findings from the program evaluation process.

In simple terms, resources represent assets and costs represent liabilities. Both resources and costs can be either monetary or non-monetary (Figure 11.1). Examples of monetary resources include tuition dollars, income from fees, additional e-learning fees, and scholarships for students, among others. Examples of non-monetary resources include building support from the larger campus (heating, cooling, electricity); technology support; library resources; student services for educational and psychological assistance; and volunteer faculty or student appointments.

Costs are also monetary or non-monetary. Monetary costs include faculty and staff salaries, testing services through outside vendors, disposable laboratory equipment fees, and learning management system fees. Some or all of these costs can be directly managed by the students (i.e., having the students pay the fees for a particular software package), or they can be paid by the institution and then recovered when students pay institutional course fees. Non-monetary costs could include problems with test-taking software that increase testing time and anxiety for students, requiring more intervention

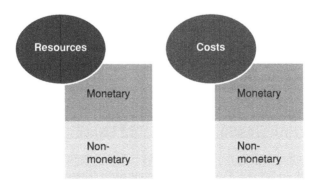

FIGURE 11.1 Institutional resources and costs.

by faculty; testing software that does not load successfully, again taking more faculty time; data entry procedures with learning management software that increase faculty work time with no increase in student learning; and faculty onboarding time in becoming familiar with multiple software programs.

There is surprisingly little literature regarding comparative and benchmarked costs associated with nursing education. Starck (2005) identified the need to understand revenue generation, though admittedly there may be little transparency about inputs (revenue generation) and outputs in higher education institutions or within specific academic units. In the absence of comparative data, the findings from systematic program evaluation can either have much greater importance or be of little relative value.

However, given the move in nursing practice and health care toward value-based purchasing and operations, this is an opportune time to categorize the components of value-based education, particularly in prelicensure programs. The data and analyses from program evaluation may make value-based education clearer than ever before. Because some of these components of value-based education will likely be either resources or costs, evaluation data can be the "light" that illuminates the relative importance of the monetary and non-monetary resources and costs within a nursing academic unit.

Start with Known Student Costs

The nursing unit administrator knows which programs and services are paid for by students via direct payment or student fees. Each of those costs can be tracked back to program evaluation data and inferences drawn from evaluation data that indicate if the costs of the programs or services directly impact student learning and success. If the evaluation plan does not provide information on concrete expenses such as standardized testing programs and the learning management system, this is an opportunity for faculty and administrators to begin collecting these data.

Identify Nonnegotiable Resources and Costs

Some programmatic requirements are resource intensive and cannot be changed. An example would be a state board of nursing–mandated 1:10 faculty-student ratio in clinical practice. Staffing clinical courses with adequate faculty to meet board requirements is a necessity. In other cases, schools include the state board licensing fee in their student benefits; if this was used as a marketing/recruitment tool, then shifting those costs to students would be nonnegotiable. Accreditation standards and state board of nursing rules and regulations are helpful in determining more nonnegotiable considerations.

Use Learning Analytics to Determine Effectiveness of Teaching Strategies and Associated Learning Expenses

Learning management systems used by colleges and universities often have learning analytic data available to the faculty users in aggregate form. These data can be used to assess specific learning strategies and see what is "worth the money" and the time. Trending reports point to even more sophisticated methods for precision learning among high school and college students in the years to come. Learning analytics will likely become part of the landscape for all prelicensure and graduate nursing students.

Maximize Resources within the Nursing Unit

On reflection, faculty may see ways that support-staff (non-faculty) can provide educational support that would free up faculty time for faculty-oriented activities. Some schools hire nonnurse coaches to help with course management duties, and others use graduate teaching assistants to augment learning experiences. Personnel costs are often by far the highest cost in any school of nursing; finding ways to use the optimum skill mix could benefit both faculty and students.

Evaluate the Outputs and Costs Associated with Licensing/ Credentialing Preparation

It is clear that first-time pass rates from RN licensure and advanced practice nursing certification examinations are of importance to many stakeholders within and outside of the educational environment. Attention, time, and money spent to increase the students' success should be carefully monitored and evaluated to that end. Faculty and students have opinions on "what really worked" as students prepared for these exams. Quality improvement studies within the nursing unit or full-scale research projects can be conducted to be sure that the energy directed in this area is useful and appropriate. Licensing and certification examinations are high-stakes testing that require reasoned, systematic evaluation of resources and costs.

Move Toward a Data-Driven Model for Systematic Evaluation

Unquestionably, data are going to be more important in the years to come, particularly because it remains difficult to adequately and effectively measure learning. One new initiative each year could be put into place to bring relevant data to the faculty and administrator for analysis. Given the emphasis on evidence-based nursing practice, one can easily imagine that a stronger emphasis on evidence-based teaching will be needed in nursing education.

AN EXAMPLE OF SUCCESSFUL ORGANIZATIONAL CHANGE

Our nursing program revised its undergraduate curriculum and transitioned to a concept-based curriculum in 2011. The process involved selecting a leader with a vision of the final product who also could focus on the details involved in each stage of the transition. The leader selected a steering committee that included experienced and new faculty to help guide the process. The primary stakeholders involved in the transition were faculty and administrators, with students as secondary stakeholders. Communication was critical in every phase of the process and included weekly emails and face-to face meetings.

Administrative support included rearranging classes to allow all faculty to be able to attend meetings each Monday. Data from benchmarking, licensure pass rates, and standardized test results were analyzed on Data Mondays—one day set aside each semester for faculty to review available data. Work groups were formed for course development and included faculty from a variety of specialties and at various stages of readiness for change. Members of the steering committee became unofficial leaders in the new work groups.

In addition to transitioning to a concept-based curriculum, faculty developed a competency-based clinical model along with focused learning activities to ensure that all students had relevant clinical experiences and met specific clinical requirements. Administration added a clinical coordinator and brought in expert nurses from local hospitals to fill clinical faculty roles, shifting costs from full-time to adjunct positions.

This transition changed the culture of the undergraduate faculty, resulting in each individual understanding and respecting the roles and expertise of other faculty members. Previous silos based on content, for example, pediatrics and mental health, were disrupted as faculty were required to more actively consult each other to teach conceptually.

SUMMARY

Leading organizational change effectively requires a clear understanding of current leadership change theories, along with a strong knowledge of the impact that systematic program assessment and evaluation can yield. Organizational decisions based on data derived from the program evaluation process can make the difference in relevant actions. Working with stakeholders is critical and requires high-level communication skills and strategies. Finally, nursing program unit resources and costs can be understood better and differently when strategic data analysis is used.

References

Bridges, W. (2009). *Managing transitions: Making the most of change* (3rd ed.). New York: NY: Perseus Publishing.

Burke, W. W. (2014). *Organization change: Theory and practice.* Los Angeles, CA: Sage.

Callery, C. A. (2012) Data-driven decision making in community colleges: An integrative model for institutional effectiveness. (Doctoral Dissertation). Retrieved from http://digitalcommons.nl.edu/diss/59

Capra, F. (1996). *The web of life.* New York, NY: Anchor Books.

Chand, S. (2015). System approach to management: Definition, features and evaluation. Retrieved from http://www.yourarticlelibrary.com/management/system-approach-to-management-definition-features-and-evaluation/27897/

Guerra-Lopez, I. (2012). The monitoring and impact evaluation process: A systemic approach to improving performance and impact. *International Journal of Environmental Science and Engineering Research, 3*(3), 80–85.

Holt, D. T., Helfrich, C. D., Hall, C. G., & Weiner, B. J. (2010). Are you ready? How health professionals can comprehensively conceptualize readiness for change. *Journal of General Internal Medicine. 25*(1), 50–55. doi: 10.1007/s11606-009-1112-8

Information Technology Leadership Academy. (2014). Organizational Change Management Readiness Guide. Retrieved from www.cio.ca.gov/opd/pdf/itla/21/OCM-FISCal-Readiness-Guide.pdf

Lee, T., & Cosgrove, T. (2014). Engaging doctors in the health care revolution. *Harvard Business Review, 92*(6), 105–111.

Lencioni, P. (2012). *The advantage: Why organizational health trumps everything else in business.* San Francisco, CA: Jossey-Bass.

Mandinach, E. B. (2012) A perfect time for data use: Using data-driven decision making to inform practice. *Educational Psychologist, 47*(2), 71–85. doi: 10.1080/00461520.2012.667064

McMillan, K., & Perron, A. (2013). Nurses amidst change: The concept of change fatigue offers an alternative perspective on organizational change. *Policy, Politics & Nursing Practice, 14*(1), 26–32. doi: 10.1177/1527154413481811

Starck, P. L. (2005). The cost of doing business in nursing education. *Journal of Professional Nursing, 21*, 183–190. doi:10.1016/j.profnurs.2005.04.007

Uhl-Bien, M., & Marion, R. (2011). Complexity leadership theory. In A. Bryman, D. Collinson, K. Grint, B. Jackson, & M. Uhl-Bien (Eds.). *The Sage handbook of leadership*. Los Angeles: Sage Publishing.

Wood, P., & Butt, G. (2014). Exploring the use of complexity theory and action research as frameworks for curriculum change. *Journal of Curriculum Studies, 46*, 676–696. doi: 10.1080/00220272.2014.921840

Yang, J., Shen, P. Q., Bourne, L., Mo, C. M. F., & Xue, X. (2011). A typology of operational approaches for stakeholder analysis and engagement: Findings from Hong Kong and Australia. *Construction Management and Economics, 29*, 145–162. doi: 10.1080/01446193.2010.521759

Examples of Completed Evaluation Plans

TABLE A.1

Completed Evaluation Plans for Faculty and Student Participation in Program Governance

Evaluation Plan Criterion: The governing organization and nursing education unit ensure representation of the nurse administrator and nursing faculty in governance activities; opportunities exist for student representation in governance activities.

Practical Nurse Program	Associate Degree Nursing Program	BSN Program	MSN Program	PhD Program
Persons Responsible: Director/faculty	*Persons Responsible:* Director/faculty	*Persons Responsible:* Administrative Advisory Committee	*Persons Responsible:* Administrative Advisory Committee	*Persons Responsible:* Administrative Advisory Committee
Expected Level of Achievement: 75% of full-time faculty will participate in college committees and activities.	*Expected Level of Achievement:* 75% of full-time faculty will participate in college committees and activities.	*Expected Level of Achievement:* Representation by all groups in governance activities as appropriate.	*Expected Level of Achievement:* Representation by all groups in governance activities as appropriate.	*Expected Level of Achievement:* Representation by all groups in governance activities as appropriate.
100% of full-time faculty will participate in faculty, departmental committees, and Nursing Advisory committee meetings.	100% of full-time faculty will participate in faculty, departmental committees, and Nursing Advisory committee meetings.			
All students given opportunity to participate in end-of-course evaluations.	All students given opportunity to participate in end-of-course evaluations.			
Student representatives from PN program will attend open session of faculty meetings.	Student representatives from ADN program will attend open session of faculty meetings.			

Timeframe for Evaluation:	Timeframe for Evaluation:	Timeframe for Evaluation:	Timeframe for Evaluation:
Annually	Annually at Retreat	Annually at Retreat	Annually at Retreat
Method for Assessment:	*Method for Assessment:*	*Method for Assessment:*	*Method for Assessment:*
Review membership list of faculty, students, and administration on Edgecombe Community College (ECC) committees. Audit faculty minutes for faculty participation. End-of-course surveys. Audit faculty minutes for student representative participation. Review end-of-course minutes.	Assessment of SON committee membership listing for nurse administrator, faculty, and student membership	Assessment of SON committee membership listing for nurse administrator, faculty, and student membership	Assessment of SON committee membership listing for nurse administrator, faculty, and student membership
Aggregate Results for This Year:	*Aggregate Results for This Year:*	*Aggregate Results for This Year:*	*Aggregate Results for This Year:*
Met. 85.7% of nursing faculty participate in college committees and activities. 100% of full-time faculty participate in faculty, end-of-course, and nursing advisory meetings.	Per Faculty Committee list for 2013–14, Dean of School of Nursing represented on Provost's Dean's Council.	Same as for BSN Program	Same as for BSN Program

Faculty schedule a computer lab for students to complete electronic end-of-semester surveys. All students given an opportunity for input. Since September of 2013 (minutes) student representatives have been available for the open session of faculty meetings with exception of June due to class/ clinical obligation. PN student (12/13 minutes and 2/14) representative was instrumental in the placement of the transition option planned for summer 2015.	Faculty schedule a computer lab for students to complete electronic end-of-semester surveys. All students given an opportunity. Since September of 2013 (minutes) student representatives have been available for the open session of faculty meetings with exception of June due to class/ clinical obligation.	Committee list in Annual Report shows evidence of faculty involvement in both SON and University committees. Students are represented on the following SON committees: Curriculum (2 BSN, 1 MSN, 1 PhD); Equity, Diversity & Inclusion (2 BSN, 1 PhD); Evaluation (2 BSN, 1 MSN); Learning Resources (2 BSN, 1 MSN); Research & Scholarship (2 BSN, 1 MSN, 1 PhD); Student Advisory Committee (9 BSN, 4 MSN, 1 PhD); Student Recruitment and Orientation (9 BSN)
Analysis and Strategies for Maintenance or Improvement: Continue plan for faculty participation in college committees. Review with Dean/ VP of Instruction other opportunities for faculty involvement.	*Analysis and Strategies for Maintenance or Improvement:* Continue plan for faculty participation in college committees. Review with Dean/ VP of Instruction other opportunities for faculty involvement.	*Analysis and Strategies for Maintenance or Improvement:* Continue to monitor.

Analysis and Strategies for Maintenance or Improvement: Continue to monitor.

Analysis and Strategies for Maintenance or Improvement: Continue to monitor.

Maintain plan for faculty participation in meetings. Part-time faculty are invited to each meeting by email and receive an electronic copy of the minutes.

Encourage participation of part-time faculty face-to-face and continue sending electronic copy. Maintain plan for student representation attending faculty meetings with input.

Student representatives from PN program will be added to end of course meetings beginning Fall 2014.

Maintain plan for faculty participation in meetings. Part-time faculty are invited to each meeting by email and receive an electronic copy of the minutes.

Encourage participation of part-time faculty face-to-face and continue sending electronic copy. Maintain plan for student representation attending faculty meetings with input.

Student representatives from ADN program will be added to end of course meetings beginning Fall 2014.

TABLE A.2

Completed Evaluation Plans for Faculty Expertise Criterion

Evaluation Plan Criterion: Faculty maintain expertise in their areas of responsibility

Practical Nurse Program	Associate Degree Nursing Program	BSN Program	MSN Program	PhD Program
Persons Responsible: Director of Nursing Programs	*Persons Responsible:* Director of Nursing Programs	*Persons Responsible:* Department Chairs	*Persons Responsible:* Department Chairs	*Persons Responsible:* Department Chairs
Expected Level of Achievement: 100% of faculty will demonstrate scholarship and evidence-based teaching and clinical practices.	*Expected Level of Achievement:* 100% of faculty will demonstrate scholarship and evidence-based teaching and clinical practices.	*Expected Level of Achievement:* Faculty (full- and part-time) maintain expertise in their areas of responsibility, and their performance reflects scholarship and evidence-based teaching and clinical practices. Expected faculty outcomes in teaching, scholarship, service, and practice are congruent with the mission, goals, and expected student outcomes.	*Expected Level of Achievement:* Same as for BSN Program.	*Expected Level of Achievement:* Same as for BSN Program.

Timeframe for Evaluation:	Timeframe for Evaluation:	Timeframe for Evaluation:	Timeframe for Evaluation:	Timeframe for Evaluation:
Annually (June)	Annually (June)	Annually	Annually	Annually
Method for Assessment:	**Method for Assessment:**	**Method for Assessment:**	**Method for Assessment:**	**Method for Assessment:**
Observation of classroom and clinical performance evaluation by Director of Nursing Programs; written performance evaluation by Director of Nursing Programs; Faculty Professional Activity Summary (PAS); and Professional Development Plan (PDP). CE table. Involvement in state initiatives for PN curriculum development; presentations.	Observation of classroom and clinical performance by Director of Nursing Programs; Written performance evaluation by Director of Nursing Programs; Faculty Professional Activity Summary (PAS); and Professional Development Plan (PDP). CE table. Involvement in state initiatives for ADN curriculum development; presentations.	Faculty document outcomes in teaching, scholarship, and service on their personnel report forms. Assessment of faculty goals, self-evaluation, peer evaluation, student evaluation, and administrative evaluation.	Same as for BSN Program.	Same as for BSN Program.
Aggregate Results for This Year:	**Aggregate Results for This Year:**	**Aggregate Results for This Year:**	**Aggregate Results for This Year:**	**Aggregate Results for This Year:**
Met. Evaluations are completed on all faculty, full-time and part-time, and are located in HR and director's offices. Timeline for evaluations needs to be more consistent with college policy.	**Met.** Evaluations are completed on all faculty, full-time and part-time, and are located in HR and director's offices. Timeline for evaluations needs to be more consistent with college policy.	Full-time faculty are evaluated annually based on job descriptions and guidelines for clinical track and tenure track performance by rank, as appropriate. Annual reports completed by	Same as for BSN program.	Same as for BSN program.

Continuing Education (CE) table indicates that full-time faculty have adequate CE on teaching methodologies.

2013–2014: Director involved in mini-CIP for the development of concept-based curriculum for PN Program.

4/14: Director presented on concept-based curriculum development to nursing program in NY.

2 full-time faculty completed MSN in 2012–2013.

Faculty nominated for Keihin Faculty Chair for 2012 and 2013.

CE table indicates that full-time faculty have adequate CE on teaching methodologies.

2013–2014: Director involved in mini-CIP for the development of concept-based curriculum for PN Program.

4/14: Director presented on concept-based curriculum development to nursing program in NY.

2 full-time faculty completed MSN in 2012–2013.

Faculty nominated for Keihin Faculty Chair for 2012 and 2013.

all faculty and used for evaluation. Evaluations located in all faculty files. Faculty outcomes regarding teaching research and service are documented in annual reports.

Faculty obtain peer evaluation of teaching; this form is located in the faculty handbook, p. 98. Student evaluations are completed online and results are shared with department heads and the individual faculty member. The procedure for administrative evaluation of faculty and report form are located in the faculty handbook, pp. 102 and 103. Procedure followed.

Analysis and Strategies for Maintenance or Improvement:

Develop calendar of events that need to be completed for evaluation purposes.

Add agenda item in each faculty meeting effective August 2014 for sharing scholarly activities faculty members are involved with.

Analysis and Strategies for Maintenance or Improvement:

Develop calendar of events that need to be completed for evaluation purposes.

Add agenda item in each faculty meeting effective August 2014 for sharing scholarly activities faculty members are involved with.

Analysis and Strategies for Maintenance or Improvement:

Suggest spreadsheet for aggregate documentation of faculty meeting teaching, service, and scholarship goals.

Analysis and Strategies for Maintenance or Improvement:

Suggest spreadsheet for aggregate documentation of faculty meeting teaching, service, and scholarship goals.

Analysis and Strategies for Maintenance or Improvement:

Suggest spreadsheet for aggregate documentation of faculty meeting teaching, service, and scholarship goals.

TABLE A.3

Completed Evaluation Plans for Assessment of Student Complaints

Evaluation Plan Criterion: Student complaints receive due process.

Practical Nurse Program	Associate Degree Nursing Program	BSN Program	MSN Program	PhD Program
Persons Responsible: Director of Nursing Programs	*Persons Responsible:* Director of Nursing Programs	*Persons Responsible:* Department Chairs	*Persons Responsible:* Department Chairs	*Persons Responsible:* Department Chairs
Expected Level of Achievement: 100% of grievances will be given due process per college policy.	*Expected Level of Achievement:* 100% of grievances will be given due process per college policy.	*Expected Level of Achievement:* 100% of complaints receive due process and show evidence of resolution.	*Expected Level of Achievement:* 100% of complaints receive due process and show evidence of resolution.	*Expected Level of Achievement:* 100% of complaints receive due process and show evidence of resolution.
Timeframe for Evaluation: With each occurrence	*Timeframe for Evaluation:* With each occurrence	*Timeframe for Evaluation:* Reported annually at retreat	*Timeframe for Evaluation:* Reported annually at retreat	*Timeframe for Evaluation:* Reported annually at retreat
Method for Assessment: Audit of grievance documentation	*Method for Assessment:* Audit of grievance documentation	*Method for Assessment:* Student Complaint Log	*Method for Assessment:* Student Complaint Log	*Method for Assessment:* Student Complaint Log

Aggregate Results for This Year:	Aggregate Results for This Year:	Aggregate Results for This Year:	Aggregate Results for This Year:
Met. 2 formal grievances were filed; documentation reflects due process and timely resolution.	3 formal complaints received from BSN students and report from Associate Dean for Undergraduate Programs to Administrative Advisory Council (dated 5/20/13) described due process and resolution. Procedure followed.	No complaints from MSN students this year.	No complaints from PhD students this year.
Analysis and Strategies for Maintenance or Improvement:	Analysis and Strategies for Maintenance or Improvement:	Analysis and Strategies for Maintenance or Improvement:	Analysis and Strategies for Maintenance or Improvement:
Audit of grievances indicate that student received due process.	Process followed. Continue to monitor.	Continue to monitor.	Continue to monitor.

Completed Evaluation Plans for Assessment of Curriculum by Faculty

Evaluation Plan Criterion: The curriculum is developed by the faculty and regularly reviewed to ensure integrity, rigor, and currency.

Practical Nurse Program	Associate Degree Nursing Program	BSN Program	MSN Program	PhD Program
Persons Responsible: Course coordinators and Faculty	*Persons Responsible:* Course coordinators and Faculty	*Persons Responsible:* Faculty and Curriculum Committee	*Persons Responsible:* Faculty and Curriculum Committee	*Persons Responsible:* Faculty and Curriculum Committee
Expected Level of Achievement: 100% of courses are evaluated for rigor and currency per semester. 100% of part-time faculty will participate in individual course team meeting and end-of-course evaluations.	*Expected Level of Achievement:* 100% of courses are evaluated for rigor and currency per semester. 100% of part-time faculty will participate in individual course team meeting and end-of-course evaluations.	*Expected Level of Achievement:* Curriculum is developed by the faculty and reviewed every 4 years by the Curriculum Committee.	*Expected Level of Achievement:* Curriculum is developed by the faculty and reviewed every 4 years by the Curriculum Committee.	*Expected Level of Achievement:* Curriculum is developed by the faculty and reviewed every 4 years by the Curriculum Committee.
Timeframe for Evaluation: Annually, following course implementation	*Timeframe for Evaluation:* Annually, following course implementation	*Timeframe for Evaluation:* Continuously and on a 4-year cycle for review	*Timeframe for Evaluation:* Continuously and on a 4-year cycle for review	*Timeframe for Evaluation:* Continuously and on a 4-year cycle for review
Method for Assessment: Audit of minutes of faculty meetings, review of course documents, end-of-course minutes	*Method for Assessment:* Audit of minutes of faculty meetings, review of course documents, end-of-course minutes	*Method for Assessment:* Syllabi, student evaluations, end-of-program evaluations, faculty evaluation of courses, and examples of student work are critiqued for further development of curriculum.	*Method for Assessment:* Syllabi, student evaluations, end-of-program evaluations, faculty evaluation of courses, and examples of student work are critiqued for further development of curriculum.	*Method for Assessment:* Syllabi, student evaluations, end-of-program evaluations, faculty evaluation of courses, and examples of student work are critiqued for further development of curriculum.

Aggregate Results for This Year: **Met.** 100% of nursing courses were reviewed in Spring 2012. 100% of nursing courses were reviewed in Fall 2013 and Spring 2014.	*Aggregate Results for This Year:* **Met.** 100% of nursing courses were reviewed in Spring 2012. 100% of nursing courses were reviewed in Fall 2013 and Spring 2014.	*Aggregate Results for This Year:* As per the published curriculum review plan, the Curriculum Committee review used syllabi, student evaluations, end-of-program evaluations, faculty evaluation of courses, and examples of student work to evaluate and critique courses. No BSN courses on the schedule to be reviewed this year and no changes in prelicensure BSN or RN-BSN curriculum made this year.	*Aggregate Results for This Year:* As per the published curriculum review plan, the Curriculum Committee reviewed used syllabi, student evaluations, end-of-program evaluations, faculty evaluation of courses, and examples of student work to evaluate and critique courses in the MSN and CRNA programs. Courses were found to be satisfactory or satisfactory with minor changes. Major curriculum changes were facilitated by the Curriculum Committee, including the discontinuation of the campus MSN Education and Administration programs, and approval of courses for the DNP program.	*Aggregate Results for This Year:* As per the published curriculum review plan, the Curriculum Committee reviewed used syllabi, student evaluations, and end-of-program evaluations, faculty evaluation of courses, and examples of student work to evaluate and critique courses in the PhD program. Courses were found to be satisfactory or satisfactory with minor changes.
Analysis and Strategies for Maintenance or Improvement: Developed template for end-of-course evaluation review beginning Fall 2013.	*Analysis and Strategies for Maintenance or Improvement:* Developed template for end-of-course evaluation review beginning Fall 2013.	*Analysis and Strategies for Maintenance or Improvement:* Continue to monitor.	*Analysis and Strategies for Maintenance or Improvement:* Continue to monitor.	*Analysis and Strategies for Maintenance or Improvement:* Continue to monitor.

TABLE A.5

Completed Evaluation Plans for Assessment of Physical Resources

Evaluation Plan Criterion: Physical resources are adequate to support the programs.

Practical Nurse Program	Associate Degree Nursing Program	BSN Program	MSN Program	PhD Program
Persons Responsible: Program Director	*Persons Responsible:* Program Director	*Persons Responsible:* Dean, Faculty, Students and Learning Resources Committee	*Persons Responsible:* Dean, Faculty, Students and Learning Resources Committee	*Persons Responsible:* Dean, Faculty, Students and Learning Resources Committee
Expected Level of Achievement: 85% or more of faculty will agree that the physical resources are adequate to support learning and achievement of PN program outcomes.	*Expected Level of Achievement:* 85% or more of faculty will agree that the physical resources are adequate to support learning and achievement of ADN program outcomes.	*Expected Level of Achievement:* Physical resources are adequate to support all programs.	*Expected Level of Achievement:* Physical resources are adequate to support all programs.	*Expected Level of Achievement:* Physical resources are adequate to support all programs.
85% of students or greater will agree that physical resources are adequate to support learning and achievement of program outcomes.	85% of students or greater will agree that physical resources are adequate to support learning and achievement of program outcomes.			

Timeframe for Evaluation:	Method for Assessment:	Aggregate Results for This Year:
Annually (April)	Faculty perceptions about physical facilities regarding size and adequacy to support teaching strategies reflected in program objectives used to develop budget. ECC Graduate surveys.	**Met.** Classroom space rated adequate for total of 100% graduates in both curricula. 66 (PN classroom), 576 square feet—15 tables and 30 chairs—classroom for PN with 20 students. Classroom equipped with white board, projector for computer, wireless Internet.
Annually (April)	Faculty perceptions about physical facilities regarding size and adequacy to support teaching strategies reflected in program objectives used to develop budget. ECC Graduate surveys.	**Met.** Classroom space rated adequate for total of 100% graduates in both curricula. 63/64 (ADN classroom) can hold 64 chairs/32 tables or total of 1,154 square feet (50 students; the most since 2012). 65 (ADN classroom), 460 square feet with 32 chairs and 16 tables—used for NUR 214 (less than 10 students).
Annually	Physical resources are evaluated by the dean's office and other resources are evaluated by the Learning Resources Committee; students evaluate resources on course and program evaluations.	The Dean and the Learning Resources Committee (LRC) evaluated resources and decided that a new simulation space should be planned and developed over the summer. Plans to include a home, pediatric, and adult care areas. The Dean named a simulation team. Also planned for the practice lab to receive updates and remodel.
Annually	Physical resources are evaluated by the dean's office and other resources are evaluated by the Learning Resources Committee; students evaluate resources on course and program evaluations.	Same as BSN Program.
Annually	Physical resources are evaluated by the dean's office and other resources are evaluated by the Learning Resources Committee; students evaluate resources on course and program evaluations.	Same as BSN Program.

1 nursing lab—680 square feet, 5 beds, 4 sinks, manikins, plus supply room and closet.	Classroom equipped with white board, projector for computer, wireless Internet.	University library funds were utilized with a total of $71,867 spent on resources for nursing.	
Student/faculty expressed concerns regarding heating and cooling system in lab.	1 nursing lab—680 square feet, 5 beds, 4 sinks, manikins, plus supply room and closet.	Student evaluations of physical resources taken from course and program evaluations rated resources between satisfied and highly satisfied.	
	Student/faculty expressed concerns regarding heating and cooling system in lab.		
Analysis and Strategies for Maintenance or Improvement:	*Analysis and Strategies for Maintenance or Improvement:*	*Analysis and Strategies for Maintenance or Improvement:*	*Analysis and Strategies for Maintenance or Improvement:*
Maintain and monitor.	Maintain and monitor.	Continue to monitor.	Continue to monitor.
Ductless heating and air system installed 5/14, which has improved temperature control.	Ductless heating and air system installed 5/14, which has improved temperature control.		

TABLE A.6

Completed Evaluation Plans for Graduate Satisfaction Criterion

Evaluation Plan Criterion: Graduate Program satisfaction: Qualitative and quantitative measures address graduates six to twelve months post-graduation

Practical Nurse Program	Associate Degree Nursing Program	BSN Program	MSN Program	PhD Program
Persons Responsible: Not specified	*Persons Responsible:* Not specified	*Persons Responsible:* Assistant Dean for Academic Affairs	*Persons Responsible:* Assistant Dean for Academic Affairs	*Persons Responsible:* Assistant Dean for Academic Affairs
Expected Level of Achievement: Graduate satisfaction with ECC nursing programs will be 85% or greater.	*Expected Level of Achievement:* Graduate satisfaction with ECC nursing programs will be 85% or greater.	*Expected Level of Achievement:* 80% of graduates will express program satisfaction.	*Expected Level of Achievement:* 80% of graduates will express program satisfaction.	*Expected Level of Achievement:* 80% of graduates will express program satisfaction.
Timeframe for Evaluation: PN graduates will be surveyed in February annually.	*Timeframe for Evaluation:* ADN and advanced placement graduates will be surveyed in December annually.	*Timeframe for Evaluation:* Annually, in March	*Timeframe for Evaluation:* Annually	*Timeframe for Evaluation:* Annually
Method for Assessment: Nursing graduate survey	*Method for Assessment:* Nursing graduate survey	*Method for Assessment:* Alumni Survey (10 months after graduation)	*Method for Assessment:* Alumni Survey (10 months after graduation)	*Method for Assessment:* Alumni Survey (10 months after graduation)

Aggregate Results for This Year:	Aggregate Results for This Year:	Aggregate Results for This Year:	Aggregate Results for This Year:	Aggregate Results for This Year:
PN 2013 graduates: 76% were very satisfied and 22.95% were satisfied with program outcomes. 78.9% of surveys returned.	ADN 2013 graduates: 55.1% were very satisfied and 49.45% were satisfied with program outcomes. 70.9% of surveys returned.	BSN Alumni survey results (per memo to faculty 4/11/14): For graduates one year after graduation, 100% of prelicensure and 100% of RN-BSN graduates were satisfied with the program (56 surveys returned for 19% response rate).	Survey of alumni showed 92% of alumni were satisfied with the program. 180 surveys sent; 7% response rate.	100% reported being either satisfied or highly satisfied with PhD program. Response rate: 63%.
Analysis and Strategies for Maintenance or Improvement:	*Analysis and Strategies for Maintenance or Improvement:*	*Analysis and Strategies for Maintenance or Improvement:*	*Analysis and Strategies for Maintenance or Improvement:*	*Analysis and Strategies for Maintenance or Improvement:*
Continue to work on methods to increase response rates.	Continue to work on methods to increase response rates.	Graduates satisfied, but need to increase sample size/response rate.	Graduates satisfied, but need to increase sample size/response rate.	Graduates satisfied, but need to increase sample size/response rate.

Adapted from Systematic Program Evaluation Plans of Edgecombe Community College Department of Nursing and University of North Carolina at Greensboro School of Nursing. Copyright Edgecombe Community College Department of Nursing, Tarboro, NC, and University of North Carolina at Greensboro School of Nursing, Greensboro, NC. Reprinted by permission of Edgecombe Community College Department of Nursing, Tarboro, NC, and University of North Carolina at Greensboro School of Nursing, Greensboro, NC.

Joint Committee on Standards for Educational Evaluation (JCSEE) Program Evaluation Standards Statements

Utility Standards

The utility standards are intended to increase the extent to which program stakeholders find evaluation processes and products valuable in meeting their needs.

- *U1, Evaluator Credibility:* Evaluations should be conducted by qualified people who establish and maintain credibility in the evaluation context.
- *U2, Attention to Stakeholders:* Evaluations should devote attention to the full range of individuals and groups invested in the program and affected by its evaluation.
- *U3, Negotiated Purposes:* Evaluation purposes should be identified and continually negotiated based on the needs of stakeholders.
- *U4, Explicit Values:* Evaluations should clarify and specify the individual and cultural values underpinning purposes, processes, and judgments.
- *U5, Relevant Information:* Evaluation information should serve the identified and emergent needs of stakeholders.
- *U6, Meaningful Processes and Products:* Evaluations should construct activities, descriptions, and judgments in ways that encourage participants to rediscover, reinterpret, or revise their understandings and behaviors.
- *U7, Timely and Appropriate Communicating and Reporting:* Evaluations should attend to the continuing information needs of their multiple audiences.
- *U8, Concern for Consequences and Influence:* Evaluations should promote responsible and adaptive use while guarding against unintended negative consequences and misuse.

Feasibility Standards

The feasibility standards are intended to increase evaluation effectiveness and efficiency.

- *F1, Project Management:* Evaluations should use effective project management strategies.
- *F2, Practical Procedures:* Evaluation procedures should be practical and responsive to the way that the program operates.
- *F3, Contextual Viability:* Evaluations should recognize, monitor, and balance the cultural and political interests and needs of individuals and groups.
- *F4, Resource Use:* Evaluations should use resources effectively and efficiently.

Propriety Standards

The propriety standards support what is proper, fair, legal, right, and just in evaluations.

- *P1, Responsive and Inclusive Orientation:* Evaluations should be responsive to stakeholders and their communities.

- *P2, Formal Agreements:* Evaluation agreements should be negotiated to make obligations explicit and take into account the needs, expectations, and cultural contexts of clients and other stakeholders.

- *P3, Human Rights and Respect:* Evaluations should be designed and conducted to protect human and legal rights, and maintain the dignity of participants and other stakeholders.

- *P4, Clarity and Fairness:* Evaluations should be understandable and fair in addressing stakeholder needs and purposes.

- *P5 Transparency and Disclosure:* Evaluations should provide complete descriptions of findings, limitations, and conclusions to all stakeholders, unless doing so would violate legal and propriety obligations.

- *P6, Conflicts of Interests:* Evaluations should openly and honestly identify and address real or perceived conflicts of interests that may compromise the evaluation.

- *P7, Fiscal Responsibility:* Evaluations should account for all expended resources and comply with sound fiscal procedures and processes.

Accuracy Standards

The accuracy standards are intended to increase the dependability and truthfulness of evaluation representations, propositions, and findings, especially those that support interpretations and judgments about quality.

- *A1, Justified Conclusions and Decisions:* Evaluation conclusions and decisions should be explicitly justified in the cultures and contexts where they have consequences.

- *A2, Valid Information:* Evaluation information should serve the intended purposes and support valid interpretations.

- *A3, Reliable Information:* Evaluation procedures should yield sufficiently dependable and consistent information for the intended uses.

- *A4, Explicit Program and Context Descriptions:* Evaluations should document programs and their contexts with appropriate detail and scope for the evaluation purposes.

- *A5, Information Management:* Evaluations should employ systematic information collection, review, verification, and storage methods.

- *A6, Sound Designs and Analyses:* Evaluations should employ technically adequate designs and analyses that are appropriate for the evaluation purposes.

- *A7, Explicit Evaluation Reasoning:* Evaluation reasoning leading from information and analyses to findings, interpretations, conclusions, and judgments should be clearly and completely documented.

- *A8, Communication and Reporting:* Evaluation communications should have adequate scope and guard against misconceptions, biases, distortions, and errors.

Evaluation Accountability Standards

The evaluation accountability standards encourage adequate documentation of evaluations and a metaevaluative perspective focused on improvement and accountability for evaluation processes and products.

- *E1, Evaluation Documentation:* Evaluations should fully document their negotiated purposes and implemented designs, procedures, data, and outcomes.

- *E2, Internal Metaevaluation:* Evaluators should use these and other applicable standards to examine the accountability of the evaluation design, procedures employed, information collected, and outcomes.

- *E3, External Metaevaluation:* Program evaluation sponsors, clients, evaluators, and other stakeholders should encourage the conduct of external metaevaluations using these and other applicable standards.

Sample Site Visit Schedule
and Resource Room Guide

Day One Site Visit Schedule

TABLE C.1

	Site Team Visitor 1	Site Team Visitor 2	Site Team Visitor 3	Site Team Visitor 4
7:45 AM	*Escorts:* Faculty A & B Pickup at hotel	*Escorts:* Faculty A & B Pickup at hotel	*Escorts:* Faculty A & B Pickup at Hotel	*Escorts:* Faculty A & B Pickup at hotel
8:00 AM	Orientation to computer and online course access (N/E 149)	Orientation to computer and online course access (N/E 149)	Orientation to computer and online course access (N/E 149)	Orientation to computer and online course access (N/E 149)
8:30 AM	Meet with Dean (N/E 150)	Meet with Dean (N/E 150)	Meet with Dean (N/E 150)	Meet with Dean (N/E 150)
9:00 AM	*Escort:* Dean Chancellor and Provost & Vice Chancellor (Chancellor's Conference Room) *Escort to CON:* Academic Staff A	*Escort:* Dean Chancellor and Provost & Vice Chancellor (Chancellor's Conference Room) *Escort to CON:* Academic Staff A	*Escort:* Dean Chancellor and Provost & Vice Chancellor (Chancellor's Conference Room) *Escort to CON:* Academic Staff A	*Escort:* Dean Chancellor and Provost & Vice Chancellor (Chancellor's Conference Room) *Escort to CON:* Academic Staff A
9:45 AM	Break	Break	Break	Break
10:00 AM	Graduate Program Director (N/E 148F)	Resource Room	Undergraduate Program Director (N/E 150) & ACCEL Coordinator (N/E 150)	Resource Room
10:30 AM	Research Director (N/E 149)	Resource Room		

Time	Activity	Time	Activity	Time	Activity	Time	Activity
11:00 AM	Orientation to Resource Room by the three directors	11:00 AM	Orientation to Resource Room by the three directors	11:00 AM	Orientation to Resource Room by the three directors	11:00 AM	Orientation to Resource Room by the three directors
Noon	Board of Visitors and Lunch	Noon	Board of Visitors and Lunch	Noon	Board of Visitors and Lunch	Noon	Board of Visitors and Lunch
1:00–4:00 PM	*Escort:* Faculty C Off-campus graduate clinical site visit Graduate student NP site visit with preceptors and students. Following this: CNL site visit with CNO and CNL site leader and student	1:00–2:00 PM	*Escort:* Faculty D Idea Lab with Director of Media Services (P5)	1:15–2:15 PM	*Escort:* Faculty D Head of Information Resources (TBD—meet in Polk Library lobby)	1:15–2:15 PM	Budget—Deputy Vice Chancellor; CON Business Manager; Dean (N/E 148B)
		2:00–2:30 PM	*Escort:* University Staff A Admissions—Director of Admissions (D135L)	2:15–3:00 PM	*Escort:* Faculty D Undergrad Classes (Research—N/E 39A)	2:30–3:15 PM	Assessment—Chair, University Assessment Committee (N/E 150)
2:30–3:30 PM	Resource Room (N/E 149)	2:30–3:30 PM	Resource Room (N/E 149)	3:00–3:30 PM	Resource Room (N/E 149)	3:00–3:30 PM	Resource Room (N/E 149)
3:45–4:45 PM	Undergraduate Student Group Meeting (N/E 151)	3:45–4:45 PM	Undergraduate Student Group Meeting (N/E 151)	3:45–4:45 PM	Undergraduate Student Group Meeting (N/E 151)	3:45–4:45 PM	Undergraduate Student Group Meeting (N/E 151)
4:30–5:00 PM	Resource Room (N/E 149)	4:45–5:00 PM	Resource Room (N/E 149)	4:45–5:00 PM	Resource Room (N/E 149)	4:45–5:00 PM	Resource Room (N/E 149)

TABLE C.2

Resource Room Guide Examples

STANDARD (Mission, Governance)

Criteria	Description	Location Unit	Location Shelf
IA	Faculty/student accomplishments (Faculty/IAS Scholarship)	A	1
	Faculty meeting minutes	A	3
IB	Faculty meeting minutes April 2009; May 18, June 3, September 8, 2009	A	3
	Faculty Handbook	A	4
	Assessment plan (Resource file)	A	1
	Undergraduate Program Committee meeting minutes May 8, 2009	A	4
	Community of interest letter (Third-Party Letter) (Resource file)	A	1
IC	College Committee minutes May 1, 2009	A	3
	Personnel Committee minutes June 4, 2009	Dean's office	
IF	Faculty meeting minutes	A	3
Other supporting documentation			
	Mission (*CON Faculty Handbook*)	A	4
	Goals (CON Strategic Planning Initiative)	A	4
	Undergraduate and Graduate Program outcomes (*CON Faculty Handbook*, pp. 8 and 13)	A	4
	Faculty outcomes (*CON Faculty Handbook* and *UW Oshkosh Personnel Handbook*)	A	4
	Professional nursing standards and guidelines:		
	Essentials of Baccalaureate Education for Professional Nursing Practice (AACN, 2008) (accordion folder)	B	4
	Graduate core curriculum content from *Essentials of Master's Education for Advanced Practice Nursing* (AACN, 1996) (accordion folder)	B	6
	Graduate core and advanced practice core from *Essentials of Master's Education for Advanced Practice Nursing* (AACN, 1996) (accordion folder)	B	6
	DNP programs: *Essentials of Doctoral Education for Advanced Nursing Practice* (AACN, 2006) (accordion folder)	B	6

TABLE C.2

Resource Room Guide Examples *(Continued)*

Criteria	Description	Unit	Shelf
		Location	
Other supporting documentation			
	Graduate programs preparing nurse practitioners from *Criteria for Evaluation of Nurse Practitioner Programs* (NTF, 2008) (NP, CNL, Nurse Educator Documentation)	B	5
	Post-baccalaureate entry programs	B	5, 6
	Additional relevant professional nursing standards and guidelines:		
	Core Competencies: Nurse Educator Clinical Nurse Leader, Nurse Practitioner	B	6
	NP, CNL, Nurse Educator Documentation	B	5
	Appointment, promotion and tenure policies or other documents defining faculty expectations:		
	UW Oshkosh Faculty and Academic Staff Handbook	A	4
	College of Nursing Faculty Handbook	A	4
	CON Personnel Committee meeting minutes	Dean's office	
	Major institutional and nursing unit reports and records for the past 3 years:		
	Faculty meeting minutes	A	3
	Strategic Planning & Initiative	A	4
	Community of interest opportunity to submit third-party comments (Resource file)	A	1
	Accrediting and regulatory agency correspondence since last accreditation review:		
	Resource file	A	1
	NP, CNL, Nurse Educator Documentation	B	5
	Catalogs, student handbooks, faculty handbooks, personnel manuals:		
	Graduate and *Undergraduate Bulletins*	Brochure stand	
	Undergraduate Student Handbook	B	4
	Graduate Student Handbook	B	5
	UW Oshkosh Faculty and Academic Staff Handbook	A	4
	Institution policies on transfer of credit: *Graduate and Undergraduate Bulletins* (Resource file)	Brochure stand	

TABLE C.2

Resource Room Guide Examples (*Continued*)

		Location	
Criteria	Description	Unit	Shelf
Other supporting documentation			
	Processes to verify that registered student in distance education is the student who participates, completes, and receives academic credit: Each student is assigned a unique ID when registering.		
	Program advertising and promotional materials directed at prospective students	Brochure stand	
	Documents that reflect decision-making (minutes, memoranda, reports)	A	3, 4
	Program policies related to formal complaints: *Undergraduate Student Handbook* *Graduate Student Handbook* *Graduate* and *Undergraduate Bulletins*	B B Brochure stand	4 5
STANDARD (Faculty)			
IIC	Dean evaluation	A	2
IID	Faculty/IAS curriculum vitae	A	1
IIE	Undergraduate preceptor evaluation forms (Preceptor Information)	B	2
	Graduate Program preceptor evaluation (Preceptor Evaluations, Faculty Evaluation of Preceptors)	B	6
IIF	CON faculty awards (Faculty Vitae)	A	1
Other supporting documentation			
	Nursing unit budget (Budget Information 2008–2010)	A	2
	Faculty and Administration: Faculty Vitae, Clinical Agencies, Curriculum and Faculty Assignments NP, CNL, Nurse Educator Documentation—NP Faculty Profiles	 A B	 1 5
	Chief Nursing Officer's vita	A	2

TABLE C.2

Resource Room Guide Examples (*Continued*)

Criteria	Description	Location Unit	Location Shelf
Other supporting documentation			
	Preceptor information:		
	NP, CNL, Nurse Educator Documentation	B	5
	Nursing 419 Clinical Synthesis: Preceptor Information; ACCEL jump drive	B	2
	Graduate Student Handbook (pp. 30–31)	B	5
	Undergraduate Student Handbook	B	4
	Current Collective Bargaining Agreement—NA		
	Policies regarding workload or teaching assignments (Faculty Handbook)	A	4
	Decision-making documents	A	2–4
STANDARD (Curriculum)			
IIIA	Evidence of how course objectives build toward specific program objectives:		
	Course binders (CON course consistency with *Baccalaureate Essentials*)	B	4
	Master's Essentials and NLN Core Competencies (NP, CNL, Nurse Educator Documentation)	B	6
IIIB	Undergraduate and graduate course consistency with respective *Baccalaureate* and *Master's Essentials:*		
	Master's Essentials and Competencies	B	6
	Undergraduate Essentials	B	4
	Graduate and undergraduate minutes re: meeting essentials and core competencies:		
	Undergraduate and Graduate Committee meeting minutes	A	3
	Core competencies	B	6
	Course syllabi (course binders)	B	1–6
	CON committee and faculty minutes	A	3
	Detailed presentation of standards and guidelines preparing students for generalist practice (Course Consistency with *Baccalaureate Essentials;* Quality Course Review)	B	4

TABLE C.2

Resource Room Guide Examples (*Continued*)

STANDARD (Curriculum)

Criteria	Description	Unit	Shelf
	Responding to change:		
	UPC meeting minutes 10/5/07	A	3
	Faculty meeting minutes 6/2/09	A	3
	Nursing 759 CNL Immersion Practicum binder	B	5
IIIC	Approval of new Undergraduate Program objectives (faculty meeting minutes, May 2009)	A	3
	Graduate practicum course building on previous clinical experience	B	4
	Course binders	B	5
	HLC DNP site visit criteria for evaluation of NP programs and DNP information (HLC Evaluation of DNP Program)	A	2
IIID	Clinical sites:		
	Clinical agencies	A	1
	NP, CNL and Nurse Educator Documentation and course binders	B	5
	Graduate student research awards	B	6
	Nursing 793 course binder	B	6
IIIE	ACCEL course changes:		
	UPC and faculty meeting minutes April and May 2009	A	3
	Course changes for ACCEL	B	4
	Criteria for evaluation of NP program reports	A	2
IIIF	Undergraduate and graduate syllabi, supplements, and evaluation (course binders)	B	1–6
IIIG	Preceptor information:		
	Undergraduate and graduate	B	2–6
	ACCEL option (flash drive in ACCEL course changes binder)	B	4
	Graduate Program Review (Resource file: assessment plans)	A	1

TABLE C.2

Resource Room Guide Examples (*Continued*)

STANDARD (Curriculum)

Criteria	Description	Unit	Shelf
		Location	
Other supporting documentation			
	Examples of student work (course binders; also in room N/E 147)	B	1–6
	Course modifications/changes based on student feedback (course binders)	B	1–6
	Current affiliation agreements (clinical agreements and contracts)	Dean's office	
	Clinical agency listing (clinical agencies binder)	A	1
	Course and faculty evaluations (undergraduate and graduate clinical and theory course evaluations)	A	5
	Documents that reflect decision-making (Undergraduate Program Committee meeting minutes binder [motions 2006–2009] and Graduate Program Committee meeting minutes	A	3
STANDARD (Program Outcomes)			
IVA	Hard copies of surveys (Program Evaluations)	A	5
	Holistic admission evaluations (Undergraduate End-of-Program Evaluations)	A	5
	Program evaluation reports (all Evaluation binders)	A	5
	Graduate Program minutes	A	3
	Programs of study (Graduate Student Handbook)	B	5
	ANP pass rates:		
	HLC Evaluation DNP Program	A	2
	NP, CNL, and NE documentation binder	B	5
	Graduate Program evaluation reports (Graduate Program Evaluation binder)	A	5
	HLC materials (HLC Evaluation DNP Program binder)	A	2
	University Assessment Plans (Resource file binder: Assessment Plans)	A	1
	Program improvement activities (Faculty Meeting Annual Reports May 2006)	A	3

TABLE C.2

Resource Room Guide Examples (*Continued*)

STANDARD (Program Outcomes)

Criteria	Description	Unit	Shelf
		Location	
IVB	Undergraduate quality review (Quality Review binder)	B	4
	Undergraduate admissions criteria:		
	Undergraduate Academic Standing Committee meeting binder	A	3
	Undergraduate Student Handbook	B	4
	Undergraduate Bulletin in brochure stand and CON website		
	Graduate preceptor information (forms, evaluation):		
	NP, CNL, and NE documentation binder	B	5
	Preceptor evaluations and faculty and student evaluations of preceptors and site binders	B	6
	Evaluation of student work:		
	Graduate course binders	B	4, 5
	Compiled statistics in accordion folder	B	6
	Graduate 1- and 5-year alumni surveys (Graduate Program evaluation binder and Alumni survey binder)	A	5
IVC	Graduate CEP rates (NP, CNL Nurse Educator documentation binder)	B	5
	Preceptor evaluation:		
	NP, CNL, and NE documentation binder	B	5
	Preceptor evaluations and faculty and student evaluations of preceptors and sites binders	B	6
IVD	Graduate Program Committee meeting minutes	A	3
	HLC documents (Overview of CON Graduate Program University accreditation and assessment for HLC 2007; HLC evaluation of DNP Program 2009 binders)	A	2
IVE	Faculty/IAS scholarship activities	A	1

TABLE C.2

Resource Room Guide Examples (*Continued*)

STANDARD (Program Outcomes)

		Location	
Criteria	**Description**	**Unit**	**Shelf**
Other supporting documentation			
	Aggregate student outcome data including:		
	Student, alumni and employer satisfaction (employer evaluation, student satisfaction binders)	A	5
	NCLEX pass rates	A	4
	Certification exam pass rates (NP, CNL, Nurse Educator documentation binder)	B	5
	Employment rates for Undergraduate and Graduate Programs (Resource file binder under Undergraduate employment rates; for graduate students in NP, CNL, and Nurse Educator documentation binder under NTF Criterion VI-c evaluation)	A B	1 1
	Summary of aggregate faculty outcome (Faculty/IAS Scholarship binder)	A	1
	Documentation of decision-making (committee meeting minutes)	A	3
	Information from formal student complaint (in Self-Study document)		

Copyright University of Wisconsin (UW) Oshkosh College of Nursing, Oshkosh, Wisconsin.
Reprinted by permission of UW Oshkosh College of Nursing, Oshkosh, Wisconsin.

← card